HAEMATOLOGY REVISION

HAEMATOLOGY REVISION

ANNABELLE S. J. BAUGHAN MRCP MRCPath
Consultant Haematologist, Ashford Hospital, Middlesex

DAVID C. LINCH MRCP
Reader in Haematology, Middlesex and University College Hospitals, London

SAMUEL J. MACHIN MRCPath
Reader in Haematology, Middlesex and University College Hospitals, London

KEITH G. PATTERSON MRCP MRCPath
Senior Lecturer in Haematology, Middlesex and University College Hospitals, London

LOUISE TILLYER MRCP MRCPath
Senior Lecturer in Haematology, London Hospital, Whitechapel, London;
Honorary Consultant Haematologist, Newham General Hospital, London

JENNIFER G. TRELEAVEN MRCP MRCPath
Consultant Haematologist, Royal Marsden Hospital, Fulham, London

CHURCHILL LIVINGSTONE
EDINBURGH LONDON MELBOURNE AND NEW YORK 1989

CHURCHILL LIVINGSTONE
Medical Division of Longman Group UK Limited

Distributed in the United States of America by Churchill Livingstone Inc., 1560 Broadway, New York, N.Y. 10036, and by associated companies, branches and representatives throughout the world.

First published 1989

ISBN 0-443-03666-7

British Library Cataloguing in Publication Data

Haematology revision.
1. Medicine. Haematology — Questions & answers
I. Baughan, Annabelle S.J. (Annabelle Sarah Jacqueline)
616.1′5′0076

Library of Congress Cataloging in Publication Data

Haematology revision/Annabelle S.J. Baughan . . . [et al.].
p. cm.
Includes index.
1. Hematology — Examinations, questions, etc. I. Baughan, Annabelle S. J.
[DNLM: 1. Hematology — examination questions. WH 18 H134]
RB 145.H245 1989
616.1′5′0076 — dc19
DNLM/DLC
for Library of Congress 88–25767
CIP

Produced by Longman Singapore Publishers (Pte) Ltd.
Printed in Singapore

PREFACE

This book contains multiple choice questions, case histories, data interpretation and pictorial slides. Each section is graded into two standards of difficulty — equivalent to the MRCP and MRCPath examinations.

Readers are encouraged to attempt both standards of question. Although many of the MRCPath cases describe rare conditions, they are not more difficult to understand or remember than the MRCP cases.

The format of the MCQs in the first section will be familiar to most examination candidates. It is only by critical assessment of your own performance that you will discover if you are too over-cautious in not following your hunches, or too confident. Read the question carefully and avoid 'reflex' answering.

When faced with a difficult slide interpretation describe to yourself what you see. This process will often trigger recognition of a condition which you have read about elsewhere.

We gratefully acknowledge the patience of our publishers, Churchill Livingstone, during the preparation of this manuscript.

London, 1989 The Authors

CONTENTS

1 MRCP Multiple Choice Questions

Each MCQ is composed of a stem followed by five statements. Any number of statements may be correct.

Assess each statement as 'true', 'false' or 'don't know'. A correct answer — either 'true' or 'false' — gains a mark. An incorrect answer results in deduction of a mark. A 'don't know' answer results in no marks being added to or subtracted from the score.

1
In liver disease

A red cell abnormalities include target cells, stomatocytes and macrocytes
B primary hepatoma may result in polycythaemia, due to ectopic production of erythropoietin
C the liver synthesises the vitamin K dependent clotting factors II, V, VII, and X
D the prothrombin time is a valuable prognostic indicator in hepatocellular failure
E alcohol excess may provoke an acute auto-immune haemolytic anaemia.

2
Blood transfusion

A 30% of cases of post-transfusion hepatitis in the UK are caused by hepatitis B virus
B in countries where malaria is endemic, all recipients of blood transfusion should be given prophylactic anti-malarial treatment
C transfusion of granulocytes from patients with chronic granulocytic leukaemia may be used therapeutically in infected neutropenic patients
D therapy with factor IX concentrate is contraindicated in hepatocellular failure and DIC
E immunosuppressed contacts of people with varicella/zoster infections should be given prophylactic fresh frozen plasma.

3
The vascular endothelial cell

A synthesises a heparin-like substance
B synthesises factor VIII:C
C releases increased amounts of prostacyclin in chronic renal failure
D produces plasminogen
E releases factor VIII:vWFag after an infusion of DDAVP.

4
Red cell morphology

A the Kleihauer cell test detects Rh positive red cells
B burr cells are typically seen in renal failure
C tear drop poikilocytes are characteristically seen in myeloma
D the degree of red cell polychromasia on blood films correlates with the reticulocyte count
E Rouleaux formation is only seen in myeloma and the connective tissue diseases.

5
In the synthesis of haem

A the enzyme δ-amino-laevulinic acid (ALA) synthetase plays a key regulatory role
B porphobilinogen is converted to uroporphyrinogen
C the final stages take place in the mitochondrion
D an abnormality in haem synthetase leads to acute intermittent porphyria
E ferrous iron is incorporated into the molecule at the final synthetic stage.

6
The normal haemoglobin molecule

A haemoglobin A_2 is formed from two α and two γ chains
B in the normal adult, haemoglobin F levels are less than 2%
C normal neonates have undetectable amounts of haemoglobin A
D haemoglobin A_{1c} is found in normal people as a result of post-synthetic modification of the β-globin chain
E reduced binding of 2, 3 diphosphoglycerate (2,3 DPG) to the haemoglobin molecule reduces its oxygen affinity.

7
Vitamin B_{12}

A most of the vitamin B_{12} in serum is in the form of methyl cobalamin
B sufficient dietary B_{12} is found in a vegan diet
C congenital lack of transcobalamin II leads to severe impairment of vitamin B_{12} metabolism
D lack of B_{12} leads to defective synthesis of myelin
E at least 1 mg of vitamin B_{12} must be given to correct a megaloblastic anaemia due to B_{12} deficiency.

8
Folic acid

A the total daily folate intake of a child should be higher than that of an adult
B active folate co-enzymes are derived from tetrahydrofolate
C folate deficiency is uncommon in coeliac disease
D megaloblastic anaemia in patients with cirrhosis is almost always due to folate deficiency
E treatment of folate deficiency in patients with malabsorption will require parenteral therapy.

9
Macrocytic anaemia

A in macrocytic anaemias the concentration of haemoglobin inside the red cell rises
B an increased mean cell volume is seen only as a late feature of liver disease associated with alcohol consumption
C megaloblastic anaemia rarely causes thrombocytopenia
D the serum iron is usually high in untreated pernicious anaemia
E serum lactate dehydrogenase (LDH) is raised in untreated megaloblastic anaemia.

10
Red cell morphology

A Howell-Jolly bodies are seen in hypersplenism
B basophilic stippling represents clumped ribosomes
C large numbers of target cells are seen in the blood of people with HbC syndromes
D in sickle cell trait approximately 10% of the red cells on the blood film will appear sickled
E between haemolytic episodes the blood film of people with G6PD deficiency will show approximately 5% spherocytes.

11
Paroxysmal nocturnal haemoglobinuria (PNH)

A the diagnostic test is Schumm's test
B the peak incidence of PNH is in the elderly
C thrombosis is a common complication
D leucopenia is a common finding
E iron deficiency anaemia occurs secondary to haematuria.

12
During pregnancy

A the red cell mass increases by approximately 25%
B the most common cause of anaemia in pregnant women in the UK is folic acid deficiency
C mild hypofibrinogenaemia is common
D a woman who needs thromboembolic prophylaxis should be given warfarin for the first six months, and then subcutaneous heparin during the last trimester
E the bone marrow is usually hypercellular.

13
In myeloma

A carpal tunnel syndrome is a recognised complication
B the white cell count at presentation is usually 2–5 $\times 10^9/1$ with 15–25% plasma cells
C the diagnosis of myeloma rests on the demonstration of a serum monoclonal paraprotein band
D thrombocytopenic bleeding is a common clinical problem
E bone X-rays are normal in 20% of cases.

14
Essential thrombocythaemia

A is a disease of young adults
B in the untreated case the blood film may show Howell-Jolly bodies, target cells and spherocytes
C gastrointestinal haemorrhage and widespread microvascular occlusion are typical clinical presentations
D splenomegaly is found in most patients
E splenectomy is the treatment of choice.

15
Blood transfusion

A all donations from blood donors in the UK are tested for syphilis, hepatitis B, cytomegalovirus antibodies and antibodies to HIV
B granulocyte transfusions must be cross-matched
C O Rh negative individuals are 'universal donors' for fresh frozen plasma
D the principal constituents of cryoprecipitate are factor VIII, fibrinogen and fibronectin
E red cells stored in optimal additive solutions must be used within three weeks of donation.

16
Sickle haemoglobin

A sickle cell disease (SCD) occurs with a frequency of 50 babies in every 100 000 births in the Afro-Caribbean community in the UK
B gallstone disease is common in SCD
C vaso-occlusive crises are seen in 10% of pregnant women with sickle cell trait
D a moderately raised plasma urea is common in SCD
E SCD may be associated with spontaneous abortions.

17
Haemoglobinopathies

A in the African variant of hereditary persistence of fetal haemoglobin (HPFH) the increased quantity of fetal (HbF) haemoglobin is distributed evenly throughout all the red cells
B one form of inherited haemoglobinopathy is manifest clinically as polycythaemia
C unstable haemoglobin variants are manifest clinically as a congenital haemolytic anaemia associated with a positive direct antiglobulin test
D the highest gene frequency of haemoglobin C is found in South Africa
E homozygous haemoglobin D disease, common in the Punjab, is virtually asymptomatic.

18
Side effects of cytotoxic drugs

A cytosine arabinoside: macrocytosis
B methotrexate: severe tissue necrosis if extravasated
C busulphan: pulmonary fibrosis
D vinca alkaloids: severe myelosuppression
E high-dose chlorambucil: haemorrhagic cystitis.

19
Haemolytic disease of the newborn (HDN)

A HDN due to anti-D antibodies is especially common in the Japanese and Chinese
B intramuscular prophylactic anti-D should be given to all Rh negative females who have inadvertently been transfused with Rh positive blood.
C prophylactic anti-D should be given to all Rh negative mothers, within 48 hours of delivery
D the severity of Rhesus D HDN is directly proportional to the titre of maternal anti-D antibodies
E affected infants with Rh D HDN who require exchange transfusions should be given ABO specific, Rh negative, concentrated red cells less than 48 hours old from donation.

20
Chronic granulocytic leukaemia

A most cases are characterised by the presence of the Philadelphia chromosome, a reciprocal translocation between chromosomes 9 and 21
B in chronic phase the blood film typically shows large numbers of neutrophils and myelocytes with only small numbers of metamyelocytes
C busulphan and hydroxyurea are first line drugs for the treatment of chronic phase disease
D allogeneic bone marrow transplantation, when appropriate, should be performed early in blast transformation of the disease
E the serum alkaline phosphatase is typically low in chronic phase CGL.

21
Blood transfusion

A the iron contained in one unit of blood administered to a person with normal iron stores will be completely excreted in six weeks
B febrile non-haemolytic blood transfusion reactions are usually caused by antibodies to granulocyte specific antigens
C citrate toxicity is seen in over 80% of patients who are transfused more than four litres of blood in 24 hours
D most delayed haemolytic transfusion reactions are due to antibodies against Rh antigens
E rapid transfusion of cold blood may cause ventricular arrythmias.

22
Macrocytic anaemia and vitamin B_{12}

A the anaemia of rheumatoid arthritis is usually macrocytic
B the Schilling test may give spurious results if performed while a patient has an untreated megaloblastic anaemia
C in Crohn's disease of the terminal ileum, an abnormally low B_{12} absorption test would correct with intrinsic factor
D approximately 90% of patients with pernicious anaemia have parietal cell antibodies in their serum
E patients with pernicious anaemia always have gastric hypochlorhydria.

23
Aplastic anaemia

A has been associated with the therapeutic use of gold
B an aetiological agent is identified in about 70% of cases
C the MCV is often raised
D the neutrophil alkaline phosphatase levels are low
E high-dose intravenous human gammaglobulin improves the blood count in approximately 50% of cases.

24
Von Willebrand's disease

A may be associated with normal factor VIII:C levels
B may be associated with an increased sensitivity to ristocetin-induced platelet aggregation
C antibodies to factor VIII:vWF develop in approximately 5% of patients
D DDAVP infusions will control bleeding episodes initially in all patients
E haemarthrosis is the most frequent presenting clinical symptom.

25
Pure red cell aplasia

A may be seen acutely in patients with sickle cell anaemia
B in adults, may be associated with myasthenia gravis
C in infants with Blackfan-Diamond syndrome, only the red cell precursors are deficient in the marrow
D corticosteroids are contraindicated in Blackfan-Diamond syndrome
E is usually accompanied by a raised reticulocyte count.

26
Infectious mononucleosis (glandular fever)

A in almost all cases causes enlargement of cervical lymph nodes
B is associated with a heterophile IgG antibody
C activated T cells are seen in the peripheral blood
D leucopenia may be seen in the first week of illness
E an increase in the cell count and protein concentration of the cerebrospinal fluid is seen in many cases.

27

The following conditions cause predominantly intravascular haemolysis

A paroxysmal nocturnal haemoglobinuria
B Rh incompatible blood transfusion
C acute reactions to oxidant drugs in G6PD deficiency
D sickle cell anaemia
E Pyruvate kinase deficiency.

28

Hereditary spherocytosis

A is the most common hereditary haemolytic anaemia in North Europeans
B in most cases red cell survival is normal after splenectomy
C is due to an abnormality of the spectrin in the red cell cytoskeleton
D spherocytes have an increased ratio of surface area to cell volume
E anaemia is usually mild.

29

Warm auto-immune haemolytic anaemia (WAIHA)

A patients on methyldopa treatment who develop a positive direct antiglobulin test (DAT) usually have IgG and complement on their red cells
B more than 50% of cases of WAIHA respond to steroid treatment
C microspherocytes are often seen in the peripheral blood film
D may be seen in association with thymoma
E blood transfusion should always be avoided.

30
Cold auto-immune haemolytic anaemia

A paroxysmal cold haemoglobinuria is associated with the Donath-Landsteiner antibody
B cold haemagglutinins with anti-i specificity are found in streptococcal infections
C paroxysmal cold haemoglobinuria is most commonly associated with acute viral infections
D the antibodies in chronic cold haemagglutinin disease are usually monoclonal
E chronic cold haemagglutinin disease usually responds to steroid therapy.

31
Thrombotic thrombocytopenic purpura (TTP) is frequently associated with

A a prolonged thrombin time
B reticulocytosis
C increased vessel wall prostacyclin release
D fragmented red cells on the blood film
E good response to steroid therapy.

32
Acetylsalicylic acid (aspirin)

A irreversibly inhibits platelet cyclo-oxygenase activity
B increases platelet cAMP activity
C increases platelet thromboxane A_2 (TXA_2) production
D inhibits vascular wall prostacyclin (PGI_2) production
E inhibits the platelet granule release reaction.

33
A prolonged bleeding time may be found in patients with

A essential thrombocythaemia
B severe anaemia with a haematocrit of < 0.20
C an overdose of warfarin
D disseminated intravascular coagulation
E hereditary antithrombin III (AT III) deficiency.

34
A prolonged thrombin time may be found in patients with

A well controlled warfarin therapy
B chronic liver disease
C raised fibrinogen degradation products (FDPs)
D acute promyelocytic leukaemia
E a raised fibrinogen level.

35
A full term normal newborn baby has

A a platelet count below $100 \times 10^9/l$
B a prolonged thrombin time
C factor VIII:C levels below 50% of adult values
D factor IX levels below 50% of adult values
E antithrombin III deficiency.

36
Long-term heparin therapy may cause

A thrombocytopenia
B osteomalacia
C alopecia
D recurrent thrombosis
E auto-immune haemolytic anaemia.

37
The following haemostatic abnormalities regularly occur in acute DIC

A increased fibrinopeptide A level
B increased antithrombin III level
C low α_2-antiplasmin level
D low factor VIII:C level
E raised plasma β-thromboglobulin.

38

Severe haemophiliacs (factor VIII:C < 0.01 iu/ml $= < 1\%$) who have received multiple infusions of factor VIII concentrate are at risk of developing

A generalised lymphadenopathy
B chronic active hepatitis
C chronic renal failure
D neutropenia
E thrombocytosis.

39

The lupus anticoagulant is associated with

A a prolonged thrombin time
B thrombocytopenia
C repeated spontaneous abortions
D a prolonged partial thromboplastin time
E positive syphilis serology.

40

Chronic idiopathic thrombocytopenic purpura (ITP) in adults is frequently associated with

A palpable splenomegaly
B permanent response to steroid therapy
C permanent response to infusion of gamma-globulin
D disseminated intravascular coagulation
E cerebral haemorrhage.

41

Glanzmann's thrombasthenia is associated with

A giant platelets on the blood film
B a defect of the platelet membrane glycoproteins IIb and IIIa
C absent platelet aggregation response to ristocetin
D autosomal dominant inheritance
E normal pathway of platelet arachidonic acid metabolism.

42
An increased incidence of venous thrombosis occurs in patients with

A polycythaemia
B multiple myeloma
C α_2-antiplasmin deficiency
D protein C deficiency
E paraplegia.

43
Physical examination in an anaemic adult may reveal the following clues to the cause of the anaemia

A brittle spoon-shaped nails in iron deficiency
B papilloedema in pernicious anaemia
C bone tenderness in aplastic anaemia
D a palpable spleen in sickle cell anaemia
E purpura in acute myeloid leukaemia.

44
The following types of anaemia are usually associated with a decreased red cell half-life

A cold haemagglutinin disease
B paroxysmal nocturnal haemoglobinuria (PNH)
C aplastic anaemia
D myelofibrosis
E hereditary spherocytosis.

45
An elevated haematocrit associated with an increased red cell mass may be found in

A renal cysts
B cholera
C erythroleukaemia
D hepatoma
E chronic bronchitis.

46
Electronic impedance blood cell counters (e.g. Coulter counters) may produce spuriously high MCV results in the following

A cold haemagglutinin disease
B pernicious anaemia
C hyperosmolar diabetic coma
D iron deficiency after treatment with parenteral iron
E rheumatoid arthritis.

47
Useful markers for distinguishing polycythaemia rubra vera from secondary polycythaemia include

A a high platelet count
B basophil leucocytosis
C splenomegaly
D neutrophilia
E a high neutrophil alkaline phosphatase score.

48
Chronic lymphocytic leukaemia

A frequently requires no treatment
B may be associated with a positive direct antiglobulin (DAT) test
C Adriamycin is the usual first line cytotoxic treatment
D a nodular pattern of marrow infiltration is associated with a better prognosis
E is always a disease of B lymphocytes.

49

A 22-year-old woman, blood group B Rh negative, is known to have anti-D antibodies during her second pregnancy. Two hours after delivery she has a massive post-partum haemorrhage

A low titre group O negative blood is suitable to restore her circulating blood volume
B intramuscular anti-D should be given within 72 hours of delivery if the baby is Rh D positive.
C in such an emergency O Rh positive blood may be transfused
D after eight units of banked blood have been transfused, coagulation factors may need to be replaced by the transfusion of 5% human albumin
E a dopamine infusion should be started to maintain blood pressure.

50

The anaemia of chronic renal failure

A is usually well tolerated
B usually responds to iron therapy
C usually responds to erythropoietin administration
D the red cells have a shortened red cell life span
E is often associated with burr cells in the blood film.

51

The following may be associated with Coombs' positive auto-immune haemolytic anaemia

A α-methyldopa (Aldomet) treatment
B intravenous penicillin treatment
C systemic lupus erythematosus (SLE)
D treatment with primaquine
E disseminated intravascular coagulation.

52

In *Plasmodium vivax* (benign tertian) malaria

A a neutrophilia is usual
B thrombocytopenia is a recognised feature

C measurement of the G6PD in the patient's red cells is a useful investigation
D the parasite is found mainly in larger red cells
E in the UK most cases are seen in travellers from Africa.

53
In a case of pancytopenia due to hypersplenism

A the bone marrow is hypocellular
B the spleen may not be clinically palpable
C a reticulocytosis is commonly present
D Gaucher's disease may be the cause
E when due to myelofibrosis, splenectomy is always beneficial.

54
In the anaemia of chronic disease

A the red cells are usually macrocytic
B the serum iron and total iron binding capacity are low
C serum ferritin is reduced
D red cell protoporphyrin is reduced
E iron utilisation is defective.

55
A dimorphic blood picture is a recognised feature of

A iron deficiency anaemia treated with iron
B pernicious anaemia after blood transfusion
C heterozygous females with G6PD deficiency
D primary sideroblastic anaemia
E renal failure on haemodialysis.

56
Iron absorption

A the principal site of absorption is the jejunum
B may be decreased by drinking tea
C may be impaired by co-existent folate deficiency
D may be excessive in β-thalassaemia
E is maximal at an alkaline pH.

57
Sideroblastic anaemia

A idiopathic sideroblastic anaemia may be improved by pyridoxine administration
B sideroblastic anaemia may be associated with a macrocytosis
C in ringed sideroblasts, the iron granules are located in the ribosomes of the erythroblast
D ringed sideroblasts are commonly found in pre-leukaemic conditions
E sideroblastic anaemia may result from over-enthusiastic iron therapy.

58
Idiopathic haemochromatosis

A may be inherited as an autosomal dominant condition
B the mainstay of treatment is chelation with desferrioxamine
C is due to a deficiency in circulating caeruloplasmin
D may predispose to the development of hepatic malignancy
E is associated with the presence of HLA B17.

59
In systemic lupus erythematosus (SLE)

A circulating coagulation inhibitors may be present
B associated thrombocytopenia is characterised by reduced numbers of bone marrow megakaryocytes
C psychiatric disorders are usually attributable to a low tissue vitamin B_{12} level
D anaemia may be due to auto-immune haemolysis
E the LE cell preparation is the most reliable way of confirming the diagnosis.

60
In chronic alcoholism

A the major cause of anaemia is malabsorption of vitamin B_{12}
B a high red cell count is usual, secondary to hypersplenism
C hypofibrinogenaemia may be found
D a high serum iron may be present
E alcohol acts as a direct suppressant of erythropoiesis.

61
Henoch-Schönlein purpura

A may be caused by an allergic hypersensitivity reaction
B the rash is due to thrombocytopenia
C is associated with gastrointestinal haemorrhage
D renal involvement may be severe, leading to irreversible renal failure
E joint symptoms are not usually prominent.

62
Amyloidosis

A may be a complication of myeloma
B is usually diagnosed by bone marrow biopsy
C may result in iron and folate deficiency
D the confirmatory histological stain is methylene blue
E is associated with chronic infective processes.

63
Heavy chain diseases

A the bone marrow always contains excess plasma cells
B the heavy chains present in the serum are polyclonal
C skeletal X-rays show discrete lytic lesions
D splenomegaly is usual in α heavy chain disease
E renal failure is the most common cause of death.

64

β thalassaemia major

A is found in Asian people
B a relative excess of α chains is present
C the haemoglobin F level is usually 10–20%
D the mainstay of treatment is blood transfusion and chelation with penicillamine
E β thalassaemia trait usually results in a mild normocytic normochromic anaemia.

65

In the α-thalassaemia syndromes

A the genetic defect lies on chromosome 9
B the condition may be clinically undetectable
C Heinz bodies are usually present in the red cells
D the finding of HbH inclusions in the red cells is pathognomonic of HbH disease
E pyridoxine may improve the anaemia in HbH disease.

66

Acute lymphoblastic leukaemia (ALL)

A the blast cells characteristically lack the enzyme terminal transferase (TdT)
B in the UK black people have a better prognosis than Caucasians
C Auer rods are commonly present in the blast cells
D disseminated intravascular coagulation (DIC) is a common complication after cytotoxic treatment of ALL
E maintenance chemotherapy should be given for at least two years.

67

Acute myeloid leukaemia (AML)

A the most common cytogenetic abnormality in de novo AML is a 9:22 translocation
B the periodic acid-Schiff (PAS) stain is usually positive
C central nervous system disease is a recognised complication

D monoblastic disease carries a better prognosis than pure myeloid disease
E is associated with prior therapy with chloramphenicol.

68
Acute lymphoblastic leukaemia (ALL)

A ALL is commonly seen as an end-stage complication of chronic lymphocytic leukaemia
B ALL has a higher relapse rate after allogeneic bone marrow transplantation than does AML
C may present as a pancytopenia
D is commonly complicated by an auto-immune haemolytic anaemia
E classical extramedullary sites of disease are the central nervous system and the ovaries.

69
Acute myeloid leukaemia (AML)

A may be a sequel to successful chemo-radiotherapy for Hodgkin's disease
B relapse is usually extramedullary
C presentation following on myelodysplastic syndrome carries a better prognosis than de novo AML
D agranular neutrophils are seen
E metabolic problems include lysozymuria and hypokalaemia.

70
Iron deficiency anaemia

A menorrhagia is the most common cause in European women
B its presence may mask the diagnosis of β-thalassaemia trait
C may rarely be associated with leucopenia
D splenomegaly and pica are well recognised findings in iron deficient adults
E may be caused by threadworms.

71

The following are true about the human major histocompatibility gene products

A Class I antigens (HLA A, B, C) are expressed on leucocytes only
B Class II antigens (Ia-like) are expressed on B cells and macrophages only
C Class I antigens mediate cell interactions in the immune response
D compatibility of Class I antigens but not Class II antigens is optimally required between donor and recipient in bone marrow transplantation
E antibodies to Class I antigens may cause resistance to platelet transfusions.

72

Iron deficiency anaemia

A when due to dietary deficiency, may be associated with a high platelet count
B is corrected more rapidly by parenteral iron therapy than by oral iron
C is commonly found in association with infestation by the fish tapeworm
D the safest iron preparation to give to a patient with a history of iron intolerance is intravenous iron dextran
E may be found as a complication of exfoliative dermatitis.

73

Prolymphocytic leukaemia

A is a variant of acute lymphoblastic leukaemia
B is as common in children as adults
C is frequently associated with massive splenomegaly
D may cause a hyperviscosity state
E the median survival is approximately seven years.

74
Neutropenia may be a feature of

A post-splenectomy states
B paroxysmal nocturnal haemoglobinuria
C glucose-6-phosphate dehydrogenase deficiency
D salmonella infections
E carbimazole therapy.

75
T lymphocytes

A comprise approximately 30% of normal peripheral blood lymphocytes
B recycle through the thymus throughout life
C have specific antigen receptors analogous to the immunoglobulin molecules
D may have a very long life span
E in viral infections there is frequently a rise in T cells of the helper/inducer (CD4+) subset.

76
Platelet transfusions

A must be cross-matched
B have a normal shelf life of two weeks
C should be given prophylactically in idopathic thrombocytopenic purpura
D may transmit cytomegalovirus (CMV)
E with long-term transfusions, most recipients will become immunised to HLA antigens.

77
A significant peripheral blood eosinophilia may be associated with

A Hodgkin's disease
B chronic lymphocytic leukaemia
C systemic lupus erythematosus
D pneumoconiosis
E Loeffler's endocarditis.

78
Burkitt's lymphoma

A is most common in SE Asia
B is a T-cell lymphoblastic lymphoma
C is associated with EBV infection
D is a low grade tumour
E frequently involves the bone marrow.

79
B lymphocytes

A originate in mammalian lymph nodes
B comprise approximately 30% of peripheral blood lymphocytes
C may express surface immunoglobulin of more than one heavy chain
D predominate in the germinal centres of the lymph node
E predominate in the peri-arteriolar cuffs of the spleen.

80
The acquired immunodeficiency syndrome

A is caused by the HTLV I virus
B is transmitted by close sexual contact only
C can be transmitted by heterosexual intercourse
D only a very small proportion of infected individuals actually develop AIDS
E the causative agent can be removed from blood products by ultrafiltration.

81
Immunoglobulins

A the major site of normal immunoglobulin production is the bone marrow
B IgM antibodies tend to react only at 37°C
C IgM is produced predominantly during a primary antibody response
D IgE antibodies mediate immediate hypersensitivity reactions

E during *Mycoplasma pneumoniae* infections, antibodies may be produced with anti-I (on red cells) specificity.

82
The following are true about HTLV I

A it is a herpes virus
B it has a high rate of infectivity
C the majority of infected individuals ultimately develop lymphoma
D HTLV I is endemic in parts of Japan and the Caribbean basin
E HTLV I lymphomas are frequently associated with hypercalcaemia.

83
Non-Hodgkin's lymphoma (NHL)

A the majority of patients have localised disease at presentation
B the histological grade has more prognostic importance than the anatomical stage
C all non-Hodgkin's lymphomas of advanced stage (III + IV) should be treated aggressively with combination chemotherapy
D patients with high grade non-Hodgkin's lymphoma who attain a complete remission should receive maintenance therapy for 2–3 years.
E the 10-year survival is higher in the high grade NHL than in the low grade NHL.

84
Graft-versus-host disease (GVHD)

A frequently occurs in recipients of syngeneic (twin) bone marrow grafts
B diarrhoea occurs in the acute form of the disease
C hepatocellular liver disease is a feature of the chronic form of the disease
D increased susceptibility to infection is a feature of GVHD
E episodes of acute GVHD usually respond to therapy with cyclosporin A.

85
Hodgkin's disease

A frequently presents with involvement of a single nodal area
B hypercalcaemia is a common complication of Hodgkin's disease
C affects the bone marrow in 35% of cases
D stage IIa disease is usually curable with local radiotherapy
E the overall 10-year survival is approximately 70%.

86
In Waldenström's macroglobulinaemia

A high levels of IgM are found in the peripheral blood
B the immunoglobulins produced may be monoclonal or polyclonal
C osteolytic bone lesions are frequently found
D hepatosplenomegaly is common
E plasmapheresis may have a role in the management of this disease.

87
Bone marrow transplantation

A may cure a large proportion of patients with severe aplastic anaemia who have matched sibling donors
B is a more effective treatment modality in children rather than young adults
C should be considered in young adults with AML and a matched donor during the first remission of their disease
D may be curative in Tay Sachs disease
E has a role in the treatment of chronic phase granulocytic leukaemia.

88
In T-cell lymproliferative disease

A mycosis fungoides may progress to the Sézary syndrome
B the finding of Sézary cells in the peripheral blood is pathognomonic of mycosis fungoides or the Sézary syndrome
C the Sézary syndrome is usually associated with hypogammaglobulinaemia
D peripheral blood eosinophilia is frequently encountered in the Sézary syndrome
E lesions of mycosis fungoides should be treated with systemic combination therapy.

89
Rhesus blood groups

A the presence of a positive direct antiglobulin test may result in false positive Rh grouping
B anti-C antibodies may cause Rh haemolytic disease of the newborn
C anti-D sensitisation may result from administration of platelet concentrate from a Rhesus positive donor
D Rhesus (D) negative patients transfused with one unit of Rhesus positive blood will invariably develop anti-D
E infants severely affected by Rh D haemolytic disease of the newborn may group as Rhesus D negative.

90
An MCV of 104 fl with normal B_{12} and folate levels may be associated with

A aplastic anaemia
B auto-immune haemolytic anaemia
C hepatic cirrhosis
D sideroblastic anaemia
E vitamin E deficiency.

91
Plasma hyperviscosity syndrome

A is seen more frequently in cases of IgA myeloma than IgG myeloma
B clinical improvement may be seen after the removal of less than 1.5 litres of plasma
C the correction of anaemia by the transfusion of packed cells should be performed before plasma exchange
D bleeding manifestations are frequently seen
E may be a presenting manifestation of monoclonal gammopathy of undetermined significance.

Answers/Comments

1 A B D

The erythrocyte abnormalities in liver disease are thought to be due to changes in the lipid constituents of the red cell membrane, secondary to changes in plasma lipids. The liver does synthesise the vitimin K dependent coagulation factors, but they are II, VII, IX (not V) and X. The constellation of acute fatty liver, acute haemolysis and hypertriglyceridaemia is known as Zieve's syndrome and may be seen after a severe alcoholic binge. However, the haemolysis is not immune-based.

2 B C D

Only 10% of post-transfusion hepatitis is thought to be due to hepatitis B; most of the rest is non-A, non-B. Granulocytes for transfusion may be prepared either from single units of donor blood, or by using a cell separator to leucapherese normal donors or patients with chronic granulocytic leukaemia (CGL). When CGL donors are used, the granulocytes must be irradiated before administration.

Factor IX concentrate is thrombogenic and should not be given in intravascular coagulation or with reduced hepatic clearance. The most useful prophylaxis against varicella/zoster is specific zoster immune globulin. Random donor fresh frozen plasma does not contain enough passive antibody to be useful except when given in vast quantities.

3 A C E

Vascular endothelial cells synthesise, store, and release into the circulation prostacyclin, PGE_1, tissue-type plasminogen activator, fibronectin, factors VIII:vWFag and VIII:vWF and small amounts of heparin-like substance. They do not synthesise or store factor VIII:C or plasminogen. After an infusion of DDAVP there is an approximately three-fold increase in the release of, and circulating levels of, factor VIII:vWFag from the vessel wall. This also occurs in patients with type I von Willebrand's disease and is a useful therapeutic approach for these patients. The release of prostacyclin is controlled by a low molecular weight plasma factor and there is evidence that this is increased in chronic renal failure. The increased release of prostacyclin contributes to the prolonged bleeding time and bleeding tendency of uraemia.

4 B D

The Kleihauer fetal cell test is used primarily to detect fetal–maternal haemorrhage in Rh negative women, but it detects cells containing fetal haemoglobin, not red cells that are Rh positive. Tear drop shaped red cells are characteristic of myelofibrosis, usually accompanied by a leucoerythroblastic blood picture. Reticulocytes, young red cells still containing RNA, have a blue–grey tinge, 'polychromasia', on conventionally stained blood films. Rouleaux formation is found in any disease state in which the erythrocyte sedimentation rate (ESR) is considerably elevated e.g. disseminated tuberculosis. When the plasma contains large quantities of protein e.g. acute phase reactants, monoclonal paraproteins etc, the red cells adhere to one another. This will be manifest as rouleaux on the blood film, and the branching chains of red cells settle faster than single red cells, thus causing a raised ESR.

5 A B C E

ALA synthetase catalyses the first and irreversible step in haem biosynthesis, the formation of δ-amino-laevulinic acid from glycine and succinyl CoA. A congenital defect in this enzyme may result in a type of sideroblastic anaemia. Porphobilinogen is converted to uroporphyrinogen and then to coproporphyrinogen. The probable abnormality in acute intermittent porphyria is a defect in uroporphyrinogen I synthetase. The incorporation of ferrous iron into the protoporphyrin ring is catalysed by haem synthetase.

6 B D

Haemoglobin A_2 consists of two α and two δ globin chains. Haemoglobin F (Fetal) consists of two α and two γ chains. Fetal haemoglobin levels fall to less than 2% of the total haemoglobin in the first 1–2 years of life. Normal neonates have significant amounts of HbA at birth, up to 50%. Total absence of HbA in a neonate indicates an homozygous hereditary defect in the haemoglobin molecule. Haemoglobin A_{1c} is formed by glycosylation of the β globin chain in circulating erythrocytes. Normal individuals have approximately 3.5% haemoglobin A_{1c}; the amount is proportional to the blood glucose level. Reduced 2,3 DPG levels lead to an increase in oxygen affinity, hence reduced oxygen delivery to the tissues.

7 A C D

Methyl cobalamin is the principal form of serum B_{12}; small amounts of 5′ deoxyadenosyl cobalamin are also found. A vegan diet has an extremely low B_{12} content. Very small amounts of B_{12} will be present in bacteria contaminating root vegetables. Transcobalamin II is responsible for most of the active transport of B_{12}; congenital absence of this protein results in a severe megaloblastic anaemia manifest in neonatal life. The mechanism whereby vitamin B_{12}

deficiency affects myelin synthesis is uncertain, but this is thought to be the aetiology of sub-acute combined degeneration of the spinal cord. As little as 0.1 μg of vitamin B_{12} will correct megaloblastic erythropoeisis in B_{12} deficiency. However, conventional treatment is with six 1 mg intramuscular injections of hydroxocobalamin to replenish body stores, repeated every three months for life in pernicious anaemia. Dietary B_{12} deficiency may be corrected by oral supplements.

8 B D

The World Health Organization recommends a daily intake of 200 μg for adults and 100 μg for children. However, weight for weight neonatal demand for folate is ten times that for adults. Newly absorbed folates undergo reduction steps in the intestine and liver, to dihydrofolate and then tetrahydrofolate. Folate deficiency is very common in coeliac disease, it is frequently the presenting manifestation. In liver disease, folate metabolism may be deranged in various ways: inadequate intake and storage, excess urinary loss, anti-folate effect of alcohol etc. In liver disease serum B_{12} levels are usually normal or increased. Even in the presence of intestinal malabsorption, a daily oral dose of 5 mg of folic acid is more than adequate treatment for folate deficiency. The duration of treatment will depend on the underlying problem.

9 D E

In macrocytic anaemias, the amount of haemoglobin within the red cell increases in proportion to the increase in cell size. The MCHC therefore remains normal. The MCV rises after only modest alcohol excess and before there is any biochemical evidence of liver disease. Thrombocytopenia and neutropenia are commonly seen in untreated megaloblastic anaemia. The fall in the neutrophil count and/or platelet count may rarely be profound. Immediately on initiating treatment for pernicious anaemia the serum iron level will fall as the iron becomes incorporated into new red cells. LDH is present in high concentration in red cells. In megaloblastic anaemias there is significant intramedullary haemolysis with subsequent release of LDH from the haemolysed erythrocytes.

10 B C

Howell-Jolly bodies are nuclear remnants and are seen as solitary erythrocyte inclusion bodies. They are found in *hyposplenism*. Basophilic stippling is found as a variant of diffuse polychromasia in many haematological disorders and in lead poisoning. Target cells have a stained centre, a pale ring, then a stained peripheral rim. This is in contrast to normal red cells which have a pale staining centre. Target cells are seen in iron deficiency, haemoglobinopathies (especially HbC) and in liver disease. With normal preparation of a fresh blood film less than 1% of the erythrocytes will be sickled in sickle trait. Between haemolytic episodes, the blood film in G6PD deficiency is normal.

11 C D

PNH is an acquired dysplastic clonal stem-cell disorder in which all three haemopoietic cell lines are unduly sensitive to the action of normal complement components. Iron deficiency anaemia is common but it is due to haemoglobinuria (not haematuria) secondary to intravascular haemolysis. The diagnostic test is Ham's acid serum haemolysis test showing an increased lytic rate of affected erythrocytes in acidified serum. (Schumm's test detects methaemalbumin.) It can occur at any age, but the peak incidence is in young adults. Patients with PNH are prone to thrombosis (often in unusual sites such as renal or portal veins) thought to be due to inappropriate platelet activation by complement and by ADP released from lysed red cells. Granulocytopenia is often seen, possibly due to premature destruction by complement.

12 A E

During pregnancy, the red cell mass increases by approximately 25% but the plasma volume increases by

50%. This net dilutional effect, maximal at 32 weeks, is the most common cause of anaemia. Normal pregnancy results in increased levels of fibrinogen. Warfarin should not be used in the first trimester as it can be teratogenic (chondrodysplasia punctata). Subcutaneous heparin should be used during the first trimester, then warfarin from about 12 to 37 weeks, then transfer back to subcutaneous heparin for easier haemostatic control at delivery to reduce the risk of maternal or fetal bleeding. Haemopoiesis is very active during pregnancy and the bone marrow is usually hypercelluler.

13 A E

Carpal tunnel syndrome may be caused by amyloidosis, which is a complication of 5–10% of cases of myeloma, particularly IgA and Bence-Jones myeloma. There is commonly a mild leucopenia at presentation but the number of circulating plasma cells is small, usually less than 5% (large numbers of circulating plasma cells are seen in the related disorder, plasma cell leukaemia). The diagnosis of myeloma may be made without a demonstrable serum monoclonal band. Equally, the presence of a monoclonal band does not necessarily mean that the patient has myeloma. A monoclonal band may be found in the serum of some healthy elderly people (benign monoclonal gammopathy) and is sometimes associated with an underlying carcinoma. Symptomatic thrombocytopenia is not a common clinical problem — the major clinical problems are bone pain, infection and renal failure. Bone radiology shows focal or diffuse lytic lesions in 60% of cases, osteoporosis alone in 20% and normal bones in 20%.

14 B C

At presentation more than 85% of patients with essential thrombocythaemia (ET) are more than 50 years old. Howell-Jolly bodies etc. are classical findings in hyposplenism, and splenic atrophy is a characteristic finding in a subgroup of patients with ET, but splenectomy is contraindicated as it will make the thrombocytosis worse. It is only considered in the very rare patient with ET who has severe secondary hypersplenism, multiple painful infarcts or myelofibrotic transformation.

15 B D

Donations are tested for syphilis, hepatitis B surface antigen and for HIV antibodies. CMV testing is not routine but some transfusion centres can supply CMV negative blood for special situations, such as transfusion of neonates and immunocompromised patients. Granulocyte concentrates are heavily contaminated with red cells and must therefore be cross-matched against the recipient's serum. Fresh frozen plasma should be of identical ABO group to the recipient; if the specific group is not available then group AB plasma is the 'universal donor' for plasma as it contains neither anti-A or anti-B antibodies. Each unit of cryoprecipitate contains approximately 80 iu of factor VIII:C, 0.25 g of fibrinogen, and 50% of the fibronectin present in the original donation. Optimal additive solutions (e.g. SAG-M — Saline Adenine Glucose Mannitol) are excellent red cell preservatives and result in a red cell shelf life of at least four weeks.

16 B E

Sickle cell disease occurs at 10 times this incidence. It is more common in the UK than phenylketonuria and congenital hypothyroidism. In common with other congenital haemolytic anaemias, pigment gallstones are common due to the increased haem turnover. Vaso-occlusive crises are virtually unknown in sickle trait except in the most exceptional circumstances e.g. a dehydrated, febrile, acidotic patient rendered hypoxic. A low plasma urea is the norm — recurrent renal tubular sickling leads to the loss of concentrating ability and reduced urea reabsorption. Maternal sickle cell disease is associated with a significant increase in the incidence of many obsteric complications, maternal and fetal.

17 A B E

There are two main types of HPFH, one with homogeneous distribution of HbF and one with heterogeneous distribution. The African variant, in which the heterozygote typically has 25% of HbF, falls in the first category. There are about 30 known congenital variants of the haemoglobin molecule which affect oxygen uptake and release. The 20 or so high-affinity variants do not easily release oxygen in the tissues, resulting in a compensatory polycythaemia. In the unstable haemoglobin variants, the direct antiglobulin test is negative. Haemolysis is due to haemoglobin precipitation within the red cell with subsequent Heinz body formation. HbC is most common in people of West African descent; the homozygous state results in mild haemolysis. Haemoglobin D has a gene frequency of 2% in the Punjab, and is associated with insignificant clinical manifestations.

18 A C

Cytosine arabinoside causes megaloblastic erythropoiesis. Other effects are immunosuppression, myelosuppression, nausea, muscle weakness and conjunctivitis with high doses. Methotrexate is not irritant; it may be given intramuscularly. Its side effects include ulceration of the mucous membranes, myelosuppression, alopecia and diarrhoea. Busulphan causes pulmonary fibrosis in a total-dose dependent manner. Other effects are prolonged myelosuppression, melanin pigmentation and premature menopause. Vinca alkaloids (vincristine, vinblastine, vindesine) are immunosuppressive but not myelosuppressive. They cause tissue necrosis on extravasation and alopecia. Vincristine causes peripheral neuropathy, ileus and constipation. Cystitis is a common side effect of high-dose cyclophosphamide, not chlorambucil. Side effects of chlorambucil include myelosuppression, immunosuppression, alopecia and hepatotoxicity.

19 E

Rhesus D HDN is virtually unknown in Japan and China as the incidence of the Rh D negative phenotype is almost 0%. Anti-D should be given to all pre-menopausal Rh negative females who have received Rh positive blood. It will usually need to be given in large *intravenous* doses — a special preparation, usually only obtainable from regional blood transfusion centres. Anti-D should be given within 48 hours of delivery but does not have to be given to those women who have delivered Rh negative babies, or who already have anti-D in their serum. The severity of haemolysis is multifactorial. It depends not only on the titre of maternal antibody but also on the rate of increase of titre during pregnancy, the subclass of antibody produced, the level of transplacental passage and other factors. Blood used for neonatal exchange transfusion should also be negative for CMV antibodies.

20 B C

The chromosomal translocation that characterises 95% of cases of CGL is between the long arms of chromosomes 9 and *22*. The exponential increase in myelocytes is faster than that of metamyelocytes so the white cell differential count classically shows neutrophil and myelocyte 'peaks'. Allogeneic marrow transplantation, in the younger patient with an HLA matched sibling donor, should be carried out in the chronic phase. The procedural mortality and the relapse rate when transplantation is carried out in blast transformation are too high to recommend transplantation at this phase of the disease. The neutrophil alkaline phosphatase score (a cytochemical technique) is reduced in CGL; the serum alkaline phosphatase is normal or slightly elevated.

21 D E

Each unit of blood contains 250 mg of iron but iron is excreted at the rate of only 1 mg daily, therefore long-term transfusion therapy in patients who are not iron deficient will lead to severe iron overload. Most febrile non-haemolytic transfusion reactions are caused by HLA-specific antibodies; antibodies to platelet-specific or granulocyte-specific antigens are responsible for only a small proportion of such reactions. Citrate toxicity is not usually seen except with massive rapid transfusion (more than one litre in ten minutes or six litres in four hours). Those most at risk are neonates, the elderly, and those with liver disease. Delayed haemolytic transfusion reactions (jaundice, anaemia, fever and arthralgia) are usually caused by an anamnestic antibody response to Rhesus antigens. Other antibodies commonly implicated are anti-Kell, Duffy and Kidd.

22 B D E

The anaemia of rheumatoid arthritis is usually normochromic and normocytic. A macrocytic anaemia due to dietary folic acid deficiency may be seen and iron deficiency may be caused by NSAID-induced gastrointestinal bleeding or dietary deficiency. In megaloblastic anaemias, the intestinal mucosa may be flattened because of folic acid or vitamin B_{12} deficiency. Performing a diagnostic Schilling test before the vitamin deficiency has been adequately treated may lead to a misleading malabsorption-type pattern of isotope excretion. In Crohn's disease of the terminal ileum the malabsorption of B_{12} will not be corrected by administration of intrinsic factor as the damaged ileum is unable to absorb the vitamin B_{12}/intrinsic factor complex. Although parietal cell antibodies are frequently found in the serum of patients with pernicious anaemia they are not specific for this disease, also being found in the sera of 10% of healthy elderly people. Intrinsic factor antibodies are far more specific for pernicious anaemia. Hypochlorhydria is a sequel of the underlying gastric atrophy.

23 A C

An idiosyncratic reaction to therapeutic gold is more commonly associated with an isolated leucopenia or thrombocytopenia. A definite aetiological agent (e.g. hepatitis A virus, chloramphenicol, benzene) is not commonly identifiable. Most cases of aplastic anaemia are idiopathic. A mild macrocytosis is commonly seen in aplastic anaemia; its pathophysiology is not clear — it may be related to underlying dyserythropoiesis. The NAP score is usually high, except when the aplasia is associated with paroxysmal nocturnal haemoglobinuria. Treatment with purified human immunoglobulin is not known to be effective in aplastic anaemia, however animal anti-lymphocyte globulin (ALG) is an important and useful treatment.

24 A B

Some patients with mild forms of type I vWD or type II vWD will have a normal factor VIII:C level. Although a decreased aggregation response to ristocetin is usually seen in vWD, patients with type IIB have an increased sensitivity even to lower concentrations of ristocetin. Unlike patients with haemophilia A, antibodies to factor VIII:vWF occur very rarely (in less than 1% of vWD patients). An infusion of DDAVP will cause an increase in factor VIII:C and factor VIII:vWF in all cases of mild and moderate type I vWD. However in other type II variants, especially type IIB, DDAVP infusions do not normalise factor VIII levels. Menorrhagia is the commonest presenting symptom in vWD, and haemarthrosis is rare.

25 A B C

Transient red cell aplasia may be seen in any of the congenital haemolytic anaemias; many cases are associated with parvovirus infection. A transient suspension of erythropoiesis due to virus infection may go unnoticed in normal people, but may become apparent in haemolytic anaemia when the red cell life span is much reduced. Red cell aplasia is known to be associated with thymomas, as is myasthenia gravis. In congenital red cell aplasia, Blackfan-Diamond syndrome, the non-erythroid marrow elements mature normally. Corticosteroid therapy is helpful in approximately 50% of patients with Blackfan-Diamond syndrome. In red cell aplasia, from whatever cause, the reticulocyte count is reduced.

26 A C D E

Cervical lymphadenopathy is almost invariable in glandular fever and is seen in the first month of illness. The heterophile antibody produced (which is detected in the Paul-Bunnell test) is an IgM antibody. Most of the atypical lymphocytes seen on the blood film in glandular fever are activated T cells. Leucopenia is common in the first week or so of the illness; it is followed by a sustained absolute lymphocytosis. Changes in the cerebrospinal fluid are seen in approximately 30% of patients tested. Serious neurological complications occur in less than 2% of all patients with glandular fever.

27 A C

In paroxysmal nocturnal haemoglobinuria the affected erythrocytes are unusually sensitive to lysis by complement. This occurs predominantly in the circulation. Transfusion of Rh incompatible blood to an individual with the relevant Rh antibody results in predominantly extravascular haemolysis i.e. a delayed haemolytic transfusion reaction with jaundice and anaemia developing 7–10 days after transfusion. Acute oxidant haemolysis in G6PD deficiency is intravascular although more chronic extravascular haemolysis can occur in some forms of G6PD deficiency. In pyruvate kinase deficiency, erythrocyte destruction occurs predominantly in the reticulo-endothelial system, as it does in sickle cell disease. In sickle cell vaso-occlusive crises there may be a transient increase in the mild degree of intravascular haemolysis.

28 A B C E

Hereditary spherocytosis is most common in North Europeans, although it has been described in most other ethnic groups. The structural abnormality is in the spectrin molecule of the cytoskeleton, resulting in the spherocytic shape of the red cell. The surface area to cell volume ratio is decreased. The haemoglobin is often normal, seldom below 9 g/dl, although transient exacerbation of the anaemia may occur with intercurrent infections. In most cases splenectomy will restore red cell survival to normal, although the spherocytic morphology remains unchanged.

29 B C D

The auto-antibody provoked in some individuals by methyldopa treatment is usually IgG alone. Approximately three-quarters of cases of WAIHA will respond to high-dose prednisone treatment, which acts by decreasing antibody production and immune adherence. In warm auto-immune haemolysis, any red cell with IgG_1 or IgG_3 or certain complement components on its membrane will be partially or completely phagocytosed by macrophages bearing appropriate receptors. If the membrane 'reseals' after partial phagocytosis, the red cell will become spherocytic. Blood transfusion in warm auto-immune haemolytic anaemia presents a number of problems — the cross-match is very difficult to interpret, and the beneficial effect of blood transfusion is often short lived. However, transfusion may be life-saving in fulminant haemolysis.

30 A C D

The Donath-Landsteiner auto-antibody is an IgG antibody which becomes maximally attached to red cells at low temperatures in the peripheral circulation. Once fixed, the antibody induces intravascular lysis by the activation of complement. This activation occurs optimally at 37°C in the central circulation. The most common cause of paroxysmal cold haemoglobinuria used to be untreated syphilis; nowadays it is usually associated with viral infections. Mycoplasma infections classically provoke cold auto-antibodies with anti-I specificity. Cold haemolysis is not a recognised feature of streptococcal infections. Chronic cold haemagglutinin disease (CHAD) is closely associated with, perhaps indistinguishable from, a lymphoid malignancy. The anti-erythrocyte antibodies in CHAD are usually monoclonal. CHAD is notoriously unresponsive to immunosuppressive or cytotoxic treatment; keeping the patient warm is usually the single most helpful therapeutic measure.

31 B D

TTP classically presents with a haemolytic anaemia, a reticulocytosis, fragmented cells on the blood film and severe thrombocytopenia due to increased platelet utilisation. The coagulation screen, including the thrombin time, is usually within the normal range and in only 10–20% of cases does disseminated intravascular coagulation secondarily occur. Histologically, platelet-fibrin aggregates are seen occluding capillaries and arterioles, and inappropriate platelet activation due to decreased vessel wall prostacyclin synthesis and release is believed to be the initiating event. Treatment regimes should include either infusion of fresh frozen plasma or vigorous plasma exchange of 3–4 litres daily. Approximately 70% of patients will respond. Corticosteroid therapy alone should not be used; responses to steroids are rare.

32 A D E

Aspirin irreversibly binds to, acetylates, and inhibits platelet cyclo-oxygenase activity. This completely blocks platelet arachidonic acid metabolism, and TXA_2 production is inhibited. The release of platelet granules (α, dense bodies and lysosomal) is dependent on TXA_2 generation, so aspirin therapy also inhibits granule release. Because platelets are unable to synthesise new enzyme, their cyclo-oxygenase activity remains inhibited for the remainder of their circulation life span. Normal platelet life span is 10–12 days. Platelet cAMP activity inhibits excessive or inappropriate platelet activation, but aspirin therapy alone has no effect on cAMP levels. Vascular endothelial cells synthesise prostacyclin from arachidonic acid via cyclo-oxygenase activity. A single dose of aspirin will inhibit vascular prostacyclin synthesis and release for only 12–24 hours before the endothelial cells are capable of synthesising new active enzyme.

33 A B D

The bleeding time is prolonged in patients with thrombocytopenia (below 70–100 $\times$ 10^9/l), in disorders of platelet function, and certain primary vessel wall defects. Thrombocytosis is usually associated with a normal or shortened bleeding time, but when due to a myeloproliferative disorder such as essential thrombocythaemia a prolonged bleeding time may be seen, due to platelet dysfunction. Severe anaemia can also affect the haemostatic process and platelet function, causing a prolonged bleeding time. Oral anticoagulation with warfarin affects only synthesis of the vitamin K dependent coagulation factors (II, VII, IX, X, proteins C and S) and has no effect on the bleeding time. Similarly AT III, which is the major natural inhibitor of thrombin and other activated coagulation factors, does not influence the bleeding time. When DIC is severe and associated with thrombocytopenia the bleeding time will be appropriately prolonged.

34 B C D E

The thrombin time measures the conversion of fibrinogen to fibrin. Patients with liver disease frequently have a prolonged thrombin time due to either reduced synthesis of fibrinogen or the synthesis of an abnormal fibrinogen molecule (dysfibrinogen). Raised levels of FDPs, which occur due to excessive fibrinolysis, e.g. in acute DIC, inhibit the action of thrombin on fibrinogen and thus may prolong the thrombin time. Acute promyelocytic leukaemia is frequently associated with acute DIC, especially during initial remission induction chemotherapy. The resulting reduced fibrinogen level and raised FDPs will prolong the thrombin time. Clottable fibrinogen levels above 6 g/l (normal range 1.5–4 g/l) will interfere with thrombin activation of fibrinogen and give a prolonged thrombin time. Warfarin therapy does not affect fibrinogen levels and has no influence on the thrombin time.

35 B D E

The haemostatic system of a newborn baby is not fully developed, mainly due to liver immaturity and partial vitamin K deficiency. Thus even the full term baby is at risk from haemorrhagic and thrombotic episodes. However the platelet count is within the normal adult range, as are the levels of factor VIII:C, which is not primarily synthesised in the liver. The thrombin time is prolonged up to twice the normal range due to decreased fibrinogen synthesis. Synthesis of factor IX and all other vitamin K dependent proteins, is also decreased by approximately 50%. The other liver coagulation factors, including the main inhibitor antithrombin III, are also decreased to varying degrees.

36 A C D

Patients who are treated with heparin, either subcutaneously as prophylaxis or intravenously, for more than 10 days are at a small risk of developing skin necrosis, thrombocytopenia, alopecia and recurrent thrombotic episodes. Osteomalacia and auto-immune haemolytic anaemia have not been reported associated with heparin therapy. Osteoporosis only develops in patients treated for 20 weeks or more but can present catastrophically with vertebral collapse. Thrombocytopenia is believed to be caused by development of specific anti-heparin antibodies which bind to the platelet membrane leading to premature platelet destruction. Heparin also occasionally causes direct platelet activation and this may precipitate the formation of in vivo platelet aggregates and the further development of thrombotic events. The most important unwanted effect of heparin therapy is bleeding.

37 A C D E

Inappropriate activation of the haemostatic mechanism is the primary pathology in acute DIC. This leads to consumption of coagulation factors (so factor VIII:C levels fall) and thrombocytopenia. As the platelets are activated they release their granular contents resulting in raised plasma β-thromboglobulin levels. Excessive thrombin activation of fibrinogen leads to release of fibrinopeptide A with resultant raised plasma levels. Secondary activation of the fibrinolytic system causes excessive plasmin generation which is initially neutralised by α_2-antiplasmin. This causes low α_2-antiplasmin levels. Antithrombin III is also consumed in an attempt to inhibit excessive factor Xa and thrombin generation. As a result of this antithrombin III levels are reduced.

38 A B D

Factor VIII concentrates are made from large pools of normal plasma and there is a risk of viral transmission of non-A non-B hepatitis, hepatitis B, and the human immunodeficiency virus (HIV). All concentrates are now screened for hepatitis B and HIV antibodies. However, haemophiliacs do develop acute hepatitis which may progress to chronic active hepatitis in a few patients. AIDS and the pre-AIDS syndromes, which include neutropenia, thrombocytopenia and generalised lymphadenopathy, occur in a significant number of haemophiliacs, due to previous exposure to non-heat treated and non-HIV screened concentrates. Chronic renal failure and thrombocytosis do not have an increased incidence in severe haemophiliacs.

39 B C D E

The lupus anticoagulant occurs in patients with SLE and related auto-immune disorders. The anticoagulant reacts with the phospholipids that provide the reactive site for factor X and V interaction, thus causing a prolonged partial thromboplastin time. The thrombin time is not prolonged. There is an increased incidence of immune-mediated thrombocytopenia, false positive syphilis serology and anti-cardiolipin antibodies due to cross reaction of the anticoagulant with platelet membrane and other phospholipids. Clinically these patients have an increased incidence of multiple thromboses, repeated abortions and intrauterine deaths.

40 NONE

ITP is an immune disorder caused by the development of auto-antibodies against platelet surface membrane. Although splenomegaly may be detected by abdominal scanning, it is rarely palpable, and if clinically enlarged another cause for the thrombocytopenia should be sought. Initial treatment with steroids or infusions of human gammaglobulin usually bring about a response, but this is only occasionally permanent. Splenectomy, however, may induce a permanent remission in 60–80% of cases. ITP is not associated with disseminated intravascular coagulation. Cerebral haemorrhage is a known complication but is rare, occurring in less than 1% of patients.

41 B E

Glanzmann's thrombasthenia is an inherited defect of platelet function with an autosomal recessive mode of inheritance. It is caused by a defect of the platelet membrane glycoproteins IIb and IIIa. This causes complete absence of platelet aggregation responses to ADP and collagen, but the primary response to ristocetin is normal. Similarly, the arachidonic acid pathway functions normally but is not activated by ADP and collagen, due to defective platelet membrane binding of these agonists. Platelet morphology appears normal on the blood film, although films made from an unanticoagulated finger-prick sample may show absence of the normal clumping of platelets.

42 A B D E

Patients who have a haematocrit above 0.50 have an increased incidence of thrombosis which rises progressively with any further increase in haematocrit. This is due to an increase in whole blood viscosity with consequent slowing and sluggishness of blood flow. In myeloma the blood viscosity may be increased by the paraprotein present in the blood. α_2-antiplasmin deficiency is associated with a bleeding tendency due to lack of plasmin inhibition leading to inappropriate fibrinolysis. Proteins S and C are vitamin K dependent proteins, and congenital deficiency of either protein predisposes to to venous thrombosis. Paraplegia causes increased venous stasis, particularly in the calf and thigh veins, and predisposes to venous thrombosis.

43 A E

The brittle spoon-shaped nails of severe iron deficiency is termed koilonychia. Angular cheilosis — splitting of the skin at the corners of the mouth — is also characteristic of iron deficiency. Papilloedema may be found in any severe anaemia. Bone tenderness is a feature of marrow infiltration with leukaemia, carcinoma, myeloma or lymphoma. The spleen is rarely palpable in adult patients with sickle cell anaemia, and these patients are usually hyposplenic due to repeated minor infarctions. The spleen may be enlarged in other sickle cell diseases, such as haemoglobin SC disease, or Sβ-thalassaemia. Purpura in acute myeloid leukaemia is a manifestation of thrombocytopenia.

44 A B D E

Red cell half-life may be measured by labelling the red cells with ^{51}Cr, reinjecting them, and taking blood samples over the following days and weeks to measure decrease in radioactivity. A rapid decline in activity implies red cell destruction or bleeding. The number of days that the radioactivity of the blood samples takes to fall to half that of the day one blood sample is termed the red cell half-life. It is usually about 27 days. Cold haemagglutinin disease, PNH and hereditary spherocytosis are all haemolytic anaemias associated with decreased red cell half-life. In aplastic anaemia the anaemia is due to marrow underproduction of red cells. The massive spleen commonly found in myelofibrosis may sequester red cells, and commonly there is an increased plasma volume contributing to the anaemia. However, the spleen may also be a site of extramedullary haemopoiesis, so isotope studies are usually performed to determine the overall contribution of the spleen to the anaemia before splenectomy is undertaken.

45 A D E

An elevated red cell mass implies a true polycythaemia. Reduction in plasma volume due to dehydration results in an increased haemoglobin and haematocrit, but the red cell volume remains normal. This is termed relative, or pseudopolycythaemia. Acute leukaemia of all types is associated with anaemia and a reduced red cell mass. Increased pressure within the renal capsule causes increased production of erythropoietin. Renal cysts and tumours may therefore result in polycythaemia. Ectopic erythropoietin-like substances may be produced by tumours. Examples are hepatoma, giant uterine fibroids, cerebellar haemangioblastoma, and carcinoma of the kidney. In chronic hypoxic chest disease increased amounts of erythropoietin are elaborated by the kidney in response to hypoxia.

46 A C

Cold haemagglutinin disease causes clumping of the red cells when the blood is allowed to cool to room temperature. These clumps of cells may be counted by the instrument as single red cells, giving rise to a false high MCV. This phenomenon may be abolished by warming the blood sample to 37°C. In hyperosmolar diabetic coma the red cells contain a high concentration of glucose in equilibrium with the plasma glucose. When the red cells are diluted in saline of normal osmolarity, preparatory to counting, water molecules diffuse rapidly into the cell, swelling it and raising the MCV. If the cells are incubated in the saline for 15 minutes then the slower-diffusing glucose molecules will equilibrate across the red cell membrane, restoring the MCV to normal. Iron deficiency is associated with a reduced MCV, and pernicious anaemia with a raised MCV. The MCV is usually normal in rheumatoid arthritis. If raised it may indicate dietary folate deficiency.

47 A B C D E

The marrow over-production of blood cells is not just confined to red cells but also involves platelets and granulocytes. All the myeloproliferative disorders (polycythaemia rubra vera, essential thrombocythaemia, chronic granulocytic leukaemia, myelofibrosis) may be associated with a basophil leucocytosis, and splenomegaly may also be found in all of them. The NAP score is raised in polycythaemia rubra vera, infections and pregnancy. It helps distinguish polycythaemia rubra vera from secondary polycythaemia.

48 A B D

Chronic lymphocytic leukaemia is frequently an incidental finding on a blood count performed in elderly patients without clinical manifestations of the disease. Some patients with the disease have an auto-immune haemolytic anaemia. The usual first line treatment is a single alkylating agent such as chlorambucil. COP (cyclophosphamide, Oncovin, prednisolone) may be used for more aggresive disease. Good prognostic factors include a nodular pattern of bone marrow infiltration, absence of splenomegaly, and a normal haemoglobin and platelet count. More than 95% of cases of CLL are of B-cell origin, but the remainder are derived from T lymphocytes.

49 A

'Universal donor' O Rh negative is kept for emergency transfusion in most blood banks, and may be used in this situation. However, if her blood group is known, then un-crossmatched blood of her group would be more appropriate. As anti-D is already present in the mother's circulation the administration of further anti-D is a fruitless exercise. Rh positive red cells will be haemolysed if transfused. Human albumin solution contains no coagulation factors, fresh frozen plasma is the appropriate replacement fluid. The administration of pressor agents such as dopamine is inappropriate. Blood volume replacement is what is required.

50 A C D E

There are a number of causes of anaemia in chronic renal failure. Failure of erythropoietin production by diseased kidneys is a major cause, and administration of cloned erythropoietin will improve the anaemia in the majority of cases. Patients with chronic renal failure have a decreased red cell life span, because of bleeding and haemolysis. Iron deficiency is unusual in chronic renal failure, though it may occur in patients who are bleeding. Burr cells are a characteristic feature of the blood film.

51 A B C

20% of patients on methyl dopa treatment for more than a year develop a positive direct antiglobulin (DAT) test. Approximately 20% of these haemolyse. Patients on large doses of penicillin with anti-penicillin antibodies may develop haemolysis. In addition to auto-immune haemolytic anaemia, patients with SLE may also develop idiopathic thrombocytopenic purpura, auto-immune neutropenia, and coagulation inhibitors. Primaquine causes a chemical oxidative (non-immune) haemolysis in G6PD deficient individuals. The haemolytic anaemia seen in DIC results from red cell destruction by fibrin strands in small blood vessels.

52 B C D

The white cell count is usually normal in *Plasmodium vivax* malaria, which may be a useful clue in distinguishing malaria from bacterial causes of a PUO. The exo-erythrocytic (liver) phase of vivax malaria is not affected by choloroquine, so will require primaquine therapy. This oxidant drug may cause haemolysis in G6PD deficient patients. Most cases of vivax malaria come from Asia, most cases of falciparum malaria come from Africa.

53 C D

The bone marrow in hypersplenism is usually hypercellular to attempt to compensate for splenic sequestration. The spleen is usually considerably enlarged when pancytopenia is present. Causes of hypersplenism include portal hypertension, myelofibrosis, chronic granulocytic leukaemia, chronic lymphocytic leukaemia, lymphoma, tropical splenomegaly, chronic infections, Felty's syndrome and

Gaucher's disease. Patients with myelofibrosis are often poor operative risks, with greatly enlarged spleens which have multiple fibrous adhesions. The spleen may also be a site of red cell production, and a careful assessment is required before splenectomy is decided upon.

54 B D E

The red cells are usually normocytic and normochromic in the anaemia of chronic disease, but may occasionally be slightly microcytic. As in iron deficiency, the serum iron is low and red cell protoporphyrin is reduced, but the total iron binding capacity is reduced. Serum ferritin is usually normal, but in active infection or inflammation its level may be increased in line with other acute phase proteins. Although iron stored in the bone marrow reticulin (macrophage) cells is normal or increased, this is not transferred to erythroblasts, which have reduced iron content.

55 A B D

After treatment of iron deficiency the population of normally haemoglobinised red cells contrasts with the older microcytic hypochromic red cells. Similarly, the macrocytic red cells of pernicious anaemia contrast with the normal size red cells that have been transfused. In sideroblastic anaemia the abnormal clones of erythroblasts in the bone marrow produce abnormally sized red cells.

56 B C D

Iron is principally absorbed in the duodenum and, to a lesser extent, the jejunum. Absorption is impaired by tea, oral chelating agents (phytates, phosphates) and alkalis. Folate deficiency may lead to malasorption of iron, secondary to abnormalities in the duodenal and jejunal epithelial lining. In β-thalassaemia major and intermedia, iron absorption is increased. The iron overload is seriously exacerbated in thalassaemia major by the blood transfusions that these patients require. Iron is maximally absorbed in the ferrous state, a low (acid) pH helps to maintain it in this state.

57 A B D

Approximately one-third of patients with either acquired or congenital sideroblastic anaemia respond to pyridoxine treatment. Sideroblastic anaemia may be associated with a normocytic, microcytic or macrocytic blood picture, and not uncommonly a dimoprhic blood picture (two populations of red cells). The iron granules in ringed sideroblasts consist of mitochondria poisoned with iron. These lie in a ring around the nucleus. Ringed sideroblasts are commonly found in the pre-leukaemic dyserythropoietic anaemias (the myelodysplastic syndromes). Pathological ringed sideroblasts are not found in simple iron overload, though marrow iron stores are increased.

58 A D

Idiopathic haemochromatosis is a genetic disorder with variable inheritance. Both dominant and recessive patterns of inheritance have been described, but it is usually autosomal recessive. The mainstay of treatment is venesection. Chelating agents such as desferrioxamine may also help to reduce the iron overload, but are very expensive and seldom used. In haemochromatosis there is no abnormality in iron carrier proteins. Caeruloplasmin is a copper-carrying protein, deficiency of which causes Wilson's disease. Cirrhosis is an invariable finding in late stages of haemochromatosis, and hepatoma develops in 10–20% of cases. There is a clear association between hereditary haemochromatosis and HLA A3, B14, and possibly B7.

59 A D

SLE is an auto-immune condition in which antibodies to many body tissues are detectable. The lupus coagulation inhibitor is found in up to 10% of patients with SLE; it is an auto-antibody which blocks the interaction of vitamin K dependent coagulation factors with platelet phospholipids. It is manifest clinically as thrombosis and spontaneous abortion. Thrombocytopenia in SLE is auto-immune in type, with normal or increased megakarycytes in the bone marrow. Vitamin B_{12} deficiency is not a feature of SLE; the psychiatric disorders are attributable to vasculitis or corticosteroid therapy. Haemolytic anaemia associated with a positive direct antiglobulin test may be seen in SLE, but more commonly 'anaemia of chronic disease' is the cause of the low haemoglobin. The LE cell preparation is positive only in 60–80% of cases of SLE. Anti-nuclear antibodies are the most sensitive test, positive in 99% of cases. The most specific test is the presence of antibodies to double-stranded DNA.

60 C D E

The anaemia of chronic alcoholism is multifactorial, but folic acid deficiency is the most common dietary cause. Alcoholics with hypersplenism and cirrhosis usually have a concomitant anaemia and normal or low red cell count. If cirrhosis is prominent, hypofibrinogenaemia may well be present. A high serum iron is present unless there is chronic blood loss. This is because alcohol increases iron absorption and decreases its utilisation in red cell manufacture. Alcohol directly suppresses erythropoiesis. Bone marrow hypoplasia may be present, with vacuolation of haemopoietic precursor cells.

61 A C D

Henoch-Schönlein purpura is thought to be due to an allergic IgA-containing immune-complex vasculitis. The allergen is often elusive; the disorder has occurred following insect bites, certain drugs and foodstuffs and as a post-streptococcal phenomenon. The rash is vasculitic, the platelet count being normal. Gastrointestinal haemorrhage may result from vasculitic lesions in the bowel. Intussusception and bowel perforation may also occur. Renal features are those of glomerulonephritis — irreversible renal failure, chronic nephritis or nephrotic syndrome may occur. Joint symptoms (polyarthralgia) are prominent, affecting about 70% of patients.

62 A C E

Amyloid is a recognised complication of myeloma and many chronic infective processes such as tuberculosis, osteomyelitis, and bronchiectasis. It is caused by the deposition in affected tissues of fibrillary material, often containing immunoglobulin light chain components. It is classically diagnosed from rectal biopsy, although it may involve many organs, including the kidney, liver, heart, skin, gastrointestinal tract, nervous and respiratory systems. If it involves the gut, iron and folate deficiency may result, secondary to malabsorption. The diagnosis is confirmed by staining biopsied material with Congo red which gives a green birefringence under a polarising microscope. (Methylene blue is a supravital stain, used in the demonstration of reticulocytes and HbH inclusions in red cells.)

63 NONE

Heavy chain diseases are very rare. They are a heterogeneous group of B-lymphoid cell proliferations, the principal common feature being the presence of a serum monoclonal protein consisting of a portion of, or the entire, heavy chain (Fc fragment) of the immunoglobulin molecule. The bone marrow may show an increase in lymphoid cells, plasma cells and eosinophils, or it may be normal. Lytic lesions are not a feature. Splenomegaly is usual in γ heavy chain disease: α heavy chain disease classically presents as a malabsorption syndrome. Renal failure may be the cause of death, but more commonly patients die of infection or bone marrow failure.

64 A B

The genetic defect in β-thalassaemia leads to an underproduction of β-globin chains in the red cells. In β-thalassaemia major, the level of HbF is raised, but usually to 60–80%. Individuals with β-thalassaemia major require lifelong blood transfusions. Excess iron has to be chelated, but with desferrioxamine. In β-thalassaemia trait, there is commonly a mild anaemia, but the haemoglobin level may be normal. However, the red cells are markedly hypochromic and microcytic.

65 B

In α-thalassaemia, the genetic defect lies on chromosome 16. Synthesis of the α-globin chain is under the control of a pair of non-allelic genes i.e. a total of four genes. There are therefore four types of α-thalassaemia, related to the number of dysfunctional genes. A four-gene dysfunction is incompatible with life (hydrops foetalis); 3-gene dysfunction results in HbH disease; 2-gene dysfunction results in a trait where the individual is clinically normal but the MCV and MCH are very low. A single-gene dysfunction is both clinically and (usually) haematologically silent. Large numbers of HbH bodies are seen in HbH disease, but small numbers may also be seen in the trait states. Pyridoxine does not improve the anaemia of HbH disease. Heinz bodies are not seen.

66 E

The blast cells in ALL are usually TdT positive. Caucasians have a better prognosis than black people — probably related to the lower frequency of T-ALL in the former. Auer rods are associated with acute myeloid leukaemia and are not found in ALL. DIC most frequently complicates the cytotoxic treatment of acute promyelocytic leukaemia when the lysis of blast cells releases thromboplastin-like granule contents. Normally, maintenance therapy is continued for two years after remission has been achieved and consolidated.

67 C

A 9:22 chromosome translocation (Philadelphia chromosome) is usually seen in chronic granulocytic leukaemia. The most common abnormalities seen in de novo AML are trisomy 8 (+8) or monosomy 7 (−7). The PAS reaction stains carbohydrate in blast cells; it is usually negative in AML, and positive in ALL. Central nervous system disease is a recognised complication of AML, particularly acute monoblastic leukaemia, although it occurs much less frequently than in ALL. Pure myeloid disease (AML M1 and M2) carries a better prognosis than disease with a monoblastic component (AML M4 and M5). Chloramphenicol is associated with subsequent development of aplastic anaemia in approximately 1 in 30 000 patients taking it, but is not thought to be associated with the development of AML.

68 B C E

Chronic lymphocytic leukaemia very rarely (< 1%) transforms into ALL. In most series ALL has a much higher relapse rate after bone marrow transplantation than AML. ALL may present haematologically as a pancytopenia alone, with blast cells absent from the peripheral blood. Autoimmune haemolytic anaemia is unusual in ALL. Central nervous system infiltration in ALL is a common and serious problem. Ovarian involvement is recognised although it is much less common than testicular involvement.

69 A D E

Approximately 1% of patients treated for Hodgkin's disease with chemo-radiotherapy develop a secondary AML. Relapse in AML is usually in the marrow, although other organs such as the CNS, skin and gums may be involved. Agranular neutrophils and other features of dysplastic granulopoiesis are frequently seen at presentation. Metabolic complications are common at presentation in AML. Lysozymuria may cause hypokalaemia by damaging renal tubules, causing a potassium leak. Rapid lysis of blast cells may result in hyperuricaemia. Hyponatraemia is common.

70 A B C

In women, menorrhagia is the commonest cause of iron deficiency, with dietary insufficiency the next most common.

Iron deficiency may mask β-thalassaemia trait, as in both conditions the haemoglobin, MCV, MCH, and MCHC are reduced. The haemoglobin A_2 level, raised in β-thalassaemia trait, may be within normal limits if the thalassaemia trait is complicated by iron deficiency. Leucopenia may be seen in association with iron deficiency; it resolves on treatment with iron. Splenomegaly and pica are found in iron deficient children, but are very unusual in adults.

71 E

The major human histocompatibility antigens are coded for in close proximity on the short arm of chromosome six. The three Class I antigens (A, B, C) are expressed on most tissues. Class II antigen expression (DR, DP, DQ) is mainly restricted to B cells, activated T cells, monocytes and myeloid progenitor cells. Class I antigens are involved in the effector functions of the cellular immune system, such as the presentation of antigen to cytotoxic (CD8+) T lymphocytes. Class II antigens serve mainly to mediate cell interactions and thus initiate and regulate the immune response. Both Class I and Class II HLA antigens act as transplantation antigens. In renal transplantation Class I antigens are most important as Class II antigens are poorly expressed on renal tissue; but in bone marrow transplantation matching of both Class I and Class II antigens is important. Platelets have low levels of Class I antigens on their surface, and in multiply transfused patients anti-HLA antibodies may be formed, giving rise to platelet resistance.

72 A E

Iron deficiency may be associated with a high platelet count in its own right, but more commonly it is a result of bleeding. Unless malabsorption is present, oral iron corrects iron deficiency as rapidly as intravenous or intramuscular iron. Classically the fish tapeworm causes deficiency of vitamin B_{12} by competitive absorption, whereas hookworm infestation leads to deficiency of iron, secondary to bleeding. Intravenous iron is absolutely contraindicated in patients with an allergic history (asthma, hay fever, eczema, etc.). It should be used with caution in patients wih rheumatoid arthritis, as it may exacerbate the arthritis. Severe anaphylactic reactions may occur during intravenous iron administration in patients with no history of atopy. Iron deficiency may be found in association with exfoliative dermatitis, when iron is lost from the skin.

73 C D

Prolymphocytic leukaemia (PLL) is a proliferation of mature lymphocytes. Although these cells have a prominent nucleolus, the nuclear chromatin pattern is condensed and the membrane phenotype is that of a relatively mature cell. Most cases are of B-cell origin although T-cell cases do occur. PLL occurs mainly in elderly patients, and typically gives rise to massive splenomegaly with very high white cell counts, especially in the T-cell variant. Extreme lymphocytoses may give rise to hyperviscosity. PLL responds poorly to treatment, and the median survival is less than three years.

74 B D E

Neutropenia may result from decreased production or increased destruction. Decreased production occurs in disorders of myeloid stem cells such as acute myeloid leukaemia, aplastic anaemia and paroxysmal nocturnal haemoglobinuria. It also occurs in other bone marrow infiltrative conditions, megaloblastic anaemia and in response to some drugs, including anti-tumour drugs and carbimazole. Increased destruction occurs with hypersplenism (not post-splenectomy) and in the presence of anti-neutrophil antibodies, the latter sometimes being induced by drugs. Many conditions cause both decreased production and increased destruction, and this includes systemic lupus erythematosus and some infections such as viral and rickettsial diseases, typhoid, brucellosis and milary TB. It should be noted that the normal range for neutrophils is lower in some racial groups, including Afro-Caribbeans.

75 C D

T lymphocytes originate in the bone marrow, and the primitive T cells then migrate to the thymus where they mature to functional, mature T cells. The majority of T cells die within the thymus and only a minority are released into the circulation. This process appears only to be important in the prenatal period and early childhood as the thymus involutes with age and thymectomy is without effect in older children and adults. Some T cells remain in the blood where they comprise approximately two-thirds of the total circulating lymphocyte population. Many of these T cells have a very long life span (memory T cells). Other T cells home to the interfollicular areas of lymph nodes and the peri-arteriolar regions of the spleen.

Although T cells have diverse phenotypes and functions they all have specific antigen receptors analogous to immunoglobulin molecules. These T-cell receptors are closely associated with the CD 3 antigen. In viral infections such as glandular fever there is typically expansion and activation of the cytotoxic/suppressor (CD8+) subset of T cells.

76 D E

Platelet transfusions are very lightly contaminated by red cells, and do not need to be cross-matched. The maximum shelf life of fresh platelets is seven days. Frozen platelets, with a greatly extended shelf life, are not yet available for routine use. The thrombocytopenia in ITP is immune-mediated, and therefore transfused platelets will also be destroyed. There is no role for prophylactic platelets in ITP; they may occasionally be given in acute haemorrhage in ITP, but are of dubious value. CMV is transmitted by transfusion of leucocytes, and platelet concentrates are commonly contaminated by leucocytes. Immunisation to HLA antigens is a common problem with long-term platelet transfusions. Such antibodies, once formed, may considerably reduce the life of transfused platelets.

77 A E

Eosinophilia is a feature of many diseases. The most common condition worldwide associated with eosinophilia is parasitic infection, particularly with metazoa and protozoa. In the UK the most common causes are dermatitis of various origins and allergic conditions such as asthma. A variety of malignant haematological diseases are associated with eosinophilia including Hodgkin's disease and the cutaneous T-cell lymphomas. Eosinophilia is not associated with chronic lymphocytic leukaemia. Eosinophilia is also commonly seen in auto-immune diseases such as polyarteritis nodosa and ulcerative colitis, but not in systemic lupus erythematosus. Loeffler's endocarditis is a rare hypereosinophilic syndrome. Eosinophilia is not a feature of the pneumoconioses.

78 C E

Burkitt's lymphoma is an aggressive malignancy of early B cells, common in East African children. It tends to involve the jaw and other extra-nodal sites such as the gut and bone marrow. In East Africa the lymphoma appears to be associated with the Epstein Barr virus (EBV genome within the malignant cells) but in sporadic cases that occur at lower frequency in other geographical areas this association with EBV is not present. Recent intensification of treatment has greatly improved the prognosis in this condition.

79 B C D E

B cells originate within the bone marrow from a common haemopoietic stem cell. In a regenerating bone marrow, B lymphoblasts (common ALL antigen+) can be readily detected. Early in B-cell development there is rearrangement of the immunoglobulin gene which contributes to antibody diversity. The clone of B cells which develops from that cell will then produce antibody with a single antigen binding specificity. The antibody is light chain restricted (either λ or κ, but not both) but more than one heavy chain isotype can be produced either over a period of time or concurrently. The B lymphocytes leave the marrow and migrate to the lymphoid tissue of the lymph nodes and spleen where they occupy the germinal centres of these organs. Some B cells predominantly remain circulating in the peripheral blood.

80 C

The acquired immunodeficiency syndrome (AIDS) is caused by the retrovirus HIV. It is transmitted by close sexual contact of heterosexual nature, although it is predominantly seen in the male homosexual population. It can also be transferred by needle-stick injuries, transfusion of blood products from infected individuals and from an infected mother to her fetus. Ultrafiltration of blood products such as factor VIII concentrate does not remove the virus, although it is largely destroyed by heat treatment. It was originally thought that only a small proportion of infected individuals developed a 'lymphadenopathy syndrome' and only a small proportion of these patients would develop AIDS. This was undoubtedly an over-optimistic estimate and it now appears that a considerable proportion of infected patients will eventually develop AIDS.

81 C D E

The major site of antibody production is within the lymphoid tissues of the lymph nodes and spleen. IgM antibodies are predominantly produced in a primary antibody response and IgG antibodies during a secondary response. IgM antibodies typically react best at temperatures below 37°C, in contrast to IgG antibodies which act rapidly at 37°C. IgA antibody levels are relatively high in tissue secretions, and IgE antibodies mediate immediate hypersensitivity reactions by their attachment to mast cells and basophils. Auto-antibodies arise in many situations and the mechanism is not well understood. Some infections give rise to high levels of auto-antibodies, a classic example being *mycoplasma pneumoniae* infection which is associated with the production of red cell antibodies with anti-I specificity.

82 D E

The human T-cell lymphotropic virus I (HTLVI) is a retrovirus endemic in certain areas, particularly Southern Japan and the Caribbean basin. It has a low rate of infectivity. Most individuals who have been infected with HTLVI (anti-HTLVI antibody positive) develop no haematological problems, but a small minority develop an aggressive lymphoma/leukaemia composed of cleaved T lymphocytes of mature CD4+ phenotype. The disease is usually widely disseminated at presentation and hypercalcaemia is common. The response to chemotherapy is very poor.

83 B E

The majority of patients with NHL have widespread disease at presentation, especially if the histology is low grade. The histological grade has more relevance to prognosis than the stage. Most cases of NHL run a slowly progressive course, although the disease is usually incurable. Patients with low grade disease only benefit from chemotherapy (even in stage III/IV) if they are symptomatic or have critical organ impairment. In the high grade lymphomas, the course is rapidly progressive if untreated, but with combination chemotherapy a considerable proportion of patients achieve complete remission and about one-third of patients are probably cured. The survival curve in the high grade NHL falls steeply in the first few years and then approximates to a plateau. The survival curve in the low grade lymphomas falls slowly but relentlessly, and beyond 10 years the survival is less than in the high grade lymphomas.

84 B D

Graft-versus-host disease occurs in many recipients of allogeneic bone marrow transplants. It has only very rarely been described in recipients of syngeneic or autologous grafts, the significance of which is not clear. In the acute form of the disease there is typically erythroderma, and occasionally exfoliation of the skin, diarrhoea and hepatocelluar liver disease. In the chronic form of the disease there are typically sclerodermatous type skin changes and obstructive liver disease. Patients with both acute and chronic graft-versus-host disease have an increased susceptibility to infection. Prophylaxis for acute GVHD is given in the form of methotrexate, cyclosporin A, or T-cell depletion of the donated graft. Cyclosporin A is not usually effective as a treatment for established GVHD, and high-dose corticosteroids are usually given in this situation.

85 A D E

Hodgkin's disease frequently presents with involvement of a single node region, and spread to other nodal areas is usually contiguous. Symptoms such as weight loss, pruritus and malaise tend to accompany advanced or histologically high grade disease and these patients may be anaemic, have a low lymphocyte count and a low serum albumin. Hypercalcaemia is rare. Despite the presence of anaemia at presentation in many patients, bone marrow involvement is present in less than 10% of cases. Stage I and IIa disease (and often IIIa disease) are usually curable with radiotherapy but for more advanced disease combination chemotherapy is necessary. The overall 10-year survival in Hodgkin's disease is approximately 70%.

86 A D E

Waldenström's macroglobulinaemia is a malignant monoclonal proliferation of plasmacytoid B lymphocytes which produce large quantities of IgM. The high levels of IgM frequently give rise to hyperviscosity syndrome. Unlike multiple myeloma, patients typically have hepatosplenomegaly and lymphadenopathy, without lytic bone lesions. Treatment is essentially palliative. Single agent chemotherapy is usually tried first, and later combination chemotherapy. Plasma exchange should be performed if hyperviscosity develops.

87 A B C E

Allogeneic bone marrow transplantation is an effective form of therapy in most patients with severe aplastic anaemia although only about 25% of patients have a matched sibling donor. The long-term results of allogeneic transplants are also superior to conventional chemotherapy in young patients (< 30 years) with AML in first remission and for patients below the age of 50 years with chronic granulocytic leukaemia (almost no long-term survivors on conventional therapy). Bone marrow transplantation may also be of value in a variety of inherited metabolic diseases where the bone marrow derived cells are the source of the missing enzyme (.e.g the mucopolysaccharidoses — not Tay Sachs disease) and in β-thalassaemia major. Allogeneic transplants are generally more successful in children than adults as the incidence of GVHD is less and the transplant related mortality reduced.

88 A D

Mycosis fungoides and Sézary syndrome represent two ends of a spectrum of lymphoproliferative disease involving the proliferation of mature CD4+ T lymphocytes. Some, but not all, patients with mycosis fungoides progress to Sézary syndrome. Patients with Sézary syndrome have circulating malignant lymphocytes which have a typically convoluted or cerebriform appearance. These cells may be seen in small numbers in mycosis fungoides without other evidence of dissemination and also in some cases of photosensitive eczema. A peripheral blood eosinophilia is often seen. The serum immunoglobulin levels are frequently raised in this disorder, in keeping with the functional helper activity of the malignant T lymphocytes. The lesions of mycosis fungoides usually respond to local therapy such as steroids, psoralens and ultraviolet light, or electron beam therapy, but disseminated Sézary's syndrome requires systemic chemotherapy. The response is often poor.

89 A B C E

If Rh grouping is performed only with an IgG anti-D in the indirect antiglobulin test then a false positive result may be obtained in patients whose red cells are already coated with IgG auto-antibody. A saline-agglutinating (IgM) anti-D reagent should be used or the direct antiglobulin test should be performed on the patient's cells. Anti-D prophylaxis is reducing the incidence of anti-D mediated haemolytic disease of the newborn, and haemolysis due to other antibodies is therefore becoming relatively more common. Red cell contamination of platelet concentrate, fresh frozen plasma or cryoprecipitate may result in anti-D sensitisation. If the administration of these Rh positive blood products to a Rh negative recipient cannot be avoided, then prophylactic anti-D should be considered. Persons transfused with Rh positive cells who do not make anti-D are termed 'non-reactors'. When all the Rh D antigenic binding sites on a baby's red cells are occupied by maternal anti-D then agglutination that should be caused by the addition of reagent anti-D may be blocked. This gives a false negative Rh grouping.

90 A B C D

The mechanism of macrocytosis in aplastic anaemia is unclear, but thought to be related to dyserythropoiesis. Young red cells are large red cells, and increased red cell destruction may result in an increase in MCV. Haemolysis may also result in folic acid deficiency. Functional liver impairment may result in macrocytosis due to abnormal red cell lipid metabolism. Target cells may be seen on the blood film. Sideroblastic anaemia may be associated with a low, normal, or high MCV.

91 A B D

The occurrence of plasma hyperviscosity syndrome not only depends on the concentration of paraprotein in the plasma, but also on the immunoglobulin class. IgM is a large molecule with a strong tendency to polymerise; IgG is smaller, with less tendency to polymerise. IgA is intermediate. The relationship between plasma viscosity and protein concentration is not linear, so the removal of small amounts of plasma may be beneficial. In addition, the larger the volume of plasma exchanged, the more normal plasma previously infused will be obtained — 'the law of diminishing returns'. The single most important determinant of whole blood viscosity is haematocrit, so whenever possible anaemia should be corrected after plasma exchange rather than before. Bleeding in hyperviscosity syndrome is due to coating of platelets by paraprotein, and interaction of paraprotein with coagulation factors. The concentration of paraprotein in monoclonal gammopathy of undetermined significance is too low to give rise to symptoms of hyperviscosity.

FURTHER READING

Question 1

McFadzean A J S, Tedd, D, Tsang K C 1958 Polycythaemia in primary carcinoma of the liver. Blood 13: 427

Rapaport S I, Ames S B, Mikkelsen S, Goodman J R 1926 Plasma clotting factors in chronic hepatocellular disease. New England Journal of Medicine 263: 278

Zieve L 1966 Hemolytic anaemia in liver disease. Medicine (Baltimore) 45: 497

Question 2

Barbara J A J, Tedder R S 1984 Viral infections transmitted by blood and its products. Clinics in Haematology 13: 693

Blatt P M, Lundblad R L, Kingdon H S, McLean G, Roberts H R 1974 Thrombogenic materials in prothrombin complex concentrates. Annals of Internal Medicine 81: 766

Question 3

Mannuci P M, Canciani M T, Rota L, Donwan B S 1981 Response of factor VIII von Willebrand factor to DDAVP in healthy subjects and patients with haemophilia A and von Willebrands disease. British Journal of Haematology 47: 283

Question 4

Dacie J V, Lewis S M 1984 Practical haematology, 6th edn. Churchill Livingstone, Edinburgh, p 62

Davey M 1979 The prevention of rhesus-isoimmunisation. Clinics in Obstetrics and Gynecology 6: 509

Kleihauer E, Braun H, Betke K 1957 Demonstration von fetalem Haemoglobin in den Erythrocyten eines blutausstrichss. Klinishe Wochenschrift 35: 637

Question 5

Rimington C 1959 Biosynthesis of haemoglobin. British Medical Bulletin 15: 19

Tschudy D P 1986 Ch 76. In: Williams, Beutler (eds) The porphyrias in hematology, 3rd edn. McGraw Hill, New York

Goldberg A 1971 Porphyrins and porphyria. In: Recent advances in haematology. Churchill, London, p 302

Question 6

Benesch R, Benesch R E 1969 Intracellular organic phosphates as regulators of oxygen release by haemoglobin. Nature 221: 618

White J M 1977 Haemoglobin structure and function: its relevance to biochemistry and medicine. In: Baum H, Gergely S (eds) Molecular aspects of medicine, vol 1, no 2

Question 7

Frenkel E P 1973 Abnormal fatty acid metabolism in peripheral nerves of patients with pernicious anaemia. Journal of Clinical Investigation 52: 1237

Hakami N, Neiman P E, Canellos G P, Lazerson J 1971 Neonatal megaloblastic anaemia due to inherited transcobalamin II deficiency in two siblings. New England Journal of Medicine 285: 1163

Hoffbrand A V, Wickremasinghe R G 1981 Megaloblastic anaemia. In: Hoffbrand A V (ed) Recent advances in haematology. Churchill Livingstone, Edinburgh, p 25

Question 8

Herbert V 1962 Minimal adult daily folate requirements. Archives of Internal Medicine 110: 649

Streiff R R 1970 Folic acid deficiency anaemia. Seminars in Haematology 7: 23

Question 9

Hoffbrand A V, Wickremasinghe R G 1981 Megaloblastic anaemia. In: Hoffbrand A V (ed) Recent advances in haematology. Churchill Livingstone, Edinburgh, p 25

Wu A, Chanarin L, Levi A J 1974 Macrocytosis of chronic alcoholism. Lancet i: 829

Question 10

Luzatto L 1975 Inherited haemolytic states: glucose 6-phosphate dehydrogenase deficiency. Clinics in Haematology 4: 83

Williams W J 1986 Examination of the blood. In: Williams W J, Beutler E, Eisler A J, Lichtman M A (eds) Hematology, 3rd edn. McGraw Hill, New York, p 9

Question 11

Sirchia G, Lewis S M 1975 Paroxysmal nocturnal haemoglobinuria. Clinics in Haematology 4(1): 199

Question 12

Jepson J H 1973 Haematological disorders in pregnancy. Clinics in Haematology 2(3)

Question 13

Durie B G M, Salmon S E 1977 Multiple myeloma, macroglobulinaemia and monoclonal gammopathies. In: Hoffbrand A V, Brain M C, Hirsh J (eds) Recent advances in haematology. Churchill Livingstone, Edinburgh, p 243

Question 14

Hardisty R M, Wolff H H 1955 Haemorrhagic thrombocythaemia: A clinical and laboratory study. British Journal of Haematology 1: 390

Question 15

Heaton A, Miripol J, Aster R et al 1984 Use of Adsol preservative solution for prolonged storage of low viscosity AS-1 red blood cells. British Journal of Haematology 57: 467

Higby D J, Barnett D 1980 Granulocyte transfusion: current status. Blood 55: 2
Watt J G 1976 Plasma fractionation. Clinics in Haematology 5: 92

Question 16

Andersen M, Went L M, MacIver J E, Dixon H G 1960 Sickle cell disease in pregnancy. Lancet ii: 516
Song Y S 1957 Hepatic lesions in sickle cell anaemia. American Journal of Pathology 33: 331
Weatherall D J (ed) 1974 Abnormal haemoglobins. Clinics in Haematology 3: No2

Question 17

Huehns E R 1970 Diseases due to abnormalities of haemoglobin sructure. Annual Review of Medicine 21: 157
Wood W G, Clegg J B, Weatherall D J 1979 Hereditary persistence of foetal haemoglogbin (HPFH) and delta-beta thalassaemia. British Journal of Haematology 43: 509

Question 18

Baughan A S J, Hughes A S B, Patterson K G, Stirling L 1985 Manual of haematology. Churchill Livingstone, Edinburgh, p 142

Question 19

Quininan J T (ed) 1971 The Rhesus problem. Clinical Obstetrics and Gynaecology 14: 494

Question 20

Goldman J M, Lu D P 1982 New approaches in chronic granulocytic leukaemia: origin prognosis and treatment. Seminars in Haematology 19: 241

Question 21

Mollison P L 1987 Blood transfusion in clinical medicine, 8th edn. Blackwell, Oxford

Question 22

Akun S N, Miller I F, Meyer L M 1969 Vitamin B_{12} absorption test. Acta Haematologica 41: 341
Hoffbrand A V (ed) 1976 Megaloblastic anaemias. Clinics in Haematology 5(3): 471

Question 23

Thomas E D (ed) 1978 Aplastic anaemia. Clinics in Haematology 7: 1

Question 24

Zimmerman T S, Meyer D 1982 Factor VIII/von Willebrand factor and the molecular basis of von Willebrand's disease. In: Colman R, Hirsh J, Marder V J et al (eds) Haemostasis and thrombosis. Lippincott, Philadelphia, p 54

Question 25

Alter B P 1980 Childhood red cell aplasia. American Journal of Pediatric Hematology and Oncology 2: 121
MacIver J E 1961 The aplastic crisis in sickle cell anaemia. Lancet i: 1086

Question 26

Carter R L 1969 Infectious mononucleosis. Blackwell Scientific Publications, Oxford

Question 27

Luzzatto L 1975 Inherited haemolytic states: glucose 6 phosphate dehydrogenase deficiency. Clinics in Haematology 4: 83
Sirchia G, Lewis S M 1975 Paroxysmal nocturnal haemoglobinuria. Clinics in Haematology 4(1): 199
Tanaka K R, Valentine W N, Miwa S 1962 Pyruvate kinase (PK) deficiency hereditary nonspherocytic hemolytic anaemia. Blood 19: 267

Question 28

Jacob H S 1972 The abnormal red cell membrane in hereditary spherocytosis: evidence for the causal role of mutant microfilaments. British Journal of Haematology 23 (suppl): 35

Schilling R F 1976 Hereditary spherocytosis. Seminars in Haematology 12: 169

Question 29

Petz L D, Garratty G 1980 Acquired immune hemolytic anaemias. Churchill Livingstone, New York

Swisher S N 1976 Immune haemolytic anaemia. Seminars in Haematology 8: 307

Question 30

Schubothe H 1966 The cold hemagglutinin diseases. Seminars in Haematology 3: 27

Worlledge S M, Rousso C 1965 Studies of the serology of paroxysmal cold haemoglobinuria (PCH) with special reference to its relationship with P blood group system. Vox Sanguinis 10: 293

Question 31

Berkowitz L R, Dalldorf F G, Blatt P M 1979 Thrombotic thrombocytopenic purpura: a pathology review. Journal of the American Medical Association 241: 1709

Bukowski R M, Hewlett J S, Reimer R R et al 1981 Therapy of thrombotic thrombocytopenic purpura: an overview. Seminars in Thrombosis and Haemostasis 7: 1

Question 32

Roth G J, Majerus P W 1975 The mechanism of the effect of aspirin on human platelets, I. Acetylation of a particulate fraction protein. Journal of Clinical Investigation 56: 624

Weiss H J, Aledort L M 1967 Impaired platelet/connective-tissue reaction in man after aspirin ingestion. Lancet ii: 495

Question 33

Dacie J V, Lewis S M 1984 Investigation of the haemostatic mechanism. In: Practical haematology, 6th edn. Churchill Livingstone, Edinburgh, p 213

Harker L A, Slichter S J 1972 The bleeding time as a screening test for evaluation of platelet function. New England Journal of Medicine 287: 155

Question 34

Dacie J V, Lewis S M 1984 Thrombin time of plasma. In: Practical haematology, 6th edn. Churchill Livingstone, Edinburgh, p 218

Question 35

Schwartz E, Gill F M 1966 Hematology of the newborn. In: Williams W J, Beutler E, Erslev A J et al (eds) Hematology, 3rd edn. McGraw Hill, New York, p 35

Question 36

Hirsh J, Gallus A S 1977 Heparin. In: Hoffbrand A V, Brain M C, Hirsh J (eds) Recent advances in haematology. Churchill Livingstone, Edinburgh, p 453

Malcolm I D, Wigmore T A 1978 Thrombocytopenia induced by low dose subcutaneous heparin. Lancet i: 444

White P W, Sadd J R, Nensel R E 1979 Thrombotic complications of heparin therapy: Including six cases of heparin induced skin necrosis. Annals of Surgery 190: 595

Question 37

Hamilton P J 1978 Disseminated intravascular coagulation: a review. Journal of Clinical Pathology 31: 609

Question 38
Hasibu U, Spero J A, Lewis J H 1977 Chronic liver dysfunction in multi-transfused haemophiliacs. Transfusion 17: 490
Kasper C K, Dietrich S L 1985 Comprehensive management of haemophilia. Clinics in Haematology 14(2): 489
Question 39
Carreras L O, Vermylen J, Spitz B, van Assche A 1981 Lupus anticoagulant and inhibition of prostacyclin formation in patients with repeated abortion, intrauterine growth retardation and intrauterine death. British Journal of Obstetrics and Gynaecology 88: 890
Schleider M A, Nachman R L, Jaffe E A, Coleman M 1976 A clinical study of the lupus anticoagulant. Blood 48: 499
Question 40
Karpatkin S 1980 Auto-immune thrombocytopenic purpura. Blood 56(3): 329
Question 41
Lusher J M, Barnhart M I 1977 Congenital disorders affecting platelets. Seminars in Thrombosis and Haemostasis 4: 123
Hardisty R M, Dormandy K M, Hutton R A 1964 Thrombasthenia: studies on 3 cases. British Journal of Haematology 10: 371
Question 42
Coon W W 1977 Epidemiology of venous thromboembolism. Annals of Surgery 186:149
Griffin J H, Evatt B, Zimmerman T S, Kleiss A J, Wideman C 1981 Deficiency of protein C in congenital thrombotic disease. Journal of Clinical Investigation 68: 1370
Question 43
Williams W J 1986 Approach to the patient. In: Hematology, 3rd edn. McGraw-Hill, New York, p 3
Question 44
Dacie J V 1960 General features of increased haemolysis. Blood picture and methods of investigation of the haemolytic anaemias. In: The haemolytic anaemias, vol 1. Churchill, London, p 1
Question 45
Erslev A J, Caro J 1983 Pathophysiology and classification of polycythaemia. Scandinavian Journal of Haematology 31: 287
Question 46
Hattersley P G, Gerard P W, Caggiano V, Nash D R 1971 Erroneous values on the model S Coulter counter due to high titre cold autoagglutinins. American Journal of Clinical Pathology 55: 442
Question 47
Lewis S M 1976 Polycythaemia vera. British Journal of Hospital Medicine 16: 125
Question 48
Galton D A G 1977 The chronic leukaemias. Clinics in Haematology 6(1)
Question 49
Mollison P L 1987 Blood transfusion in clinical medicine, 8th edn. Blackwell, Oxford
Question 50
Erslev A J 1970 Anaemia of chronic renal disease. Archives of Internal Medicine 126: 774
Question 51
Rosse W F 1981 The acquired haemolytic anaemias. In: Hoffbrand A V, Lewis S M (eds) Postgraduate haematology, 2nd edn. Heinemann, London, p 229

Question 52

Perrin L H, Mackey L J, Miescher P A 1982 The hematolgoy of malaria in man. Seminars in Haematology 19: 70

Question 53

Crosby W H 1962 Hypersplenism. Annual Review in Medicine 13: 127

Question 54

Cartwright G E 1966 The anaemia of chronic disorders. Seminars in Haematology 3: 351

Question 55

Bessman J D, Johnson R K 1975 Erythrocyte volume distribution in normal and abnormal subjects. Blood 46: 369

Question 56

Jacobs A 1970 Digestive factors in iron absorption. Progress in Gastroenterology 11: 221

Question 57

Hines J D, Grasso J A 1970 The sideroblastic anaemias. Seminars in Haematology 7: 86

Question 58

Edwards C Q, Carroll M, Bray P, Cartwright G E 1977 Hereditary hemochromatosis. New England Journal of Medicine 297: 7

Finch S C, Finch C A 1955 Idiopathic hemochromatosis, an iron storage disease. Medicine (Baltimore) 32: 381

Question 59

Bennett R, Hughes G R V, Bywaters E G L, Holt P J L 1972 Neuropsychiatric problems in systemic lupus erythematosus. British Medical Journal 4: 342

Burkhardt R 1965 The bone marrow in systemic lupus erythematosus. Seminars in Haematology 2: 29

Dubois E L 1952 Acquired haemolytic anaemia as a presenting feature of systemic lupus erythematosus. American Journal of Medicine 12: 197

Hughes G R V 1971 Significance of anti-DNA antibodies in SLE. Lancet ii: 861

Question 60

Herbert V (ed) 1980 Hematologic complications of alcoholism. Seminars in Hematology 17 (i) (ii)

McCurdy P R, Rath C E 1980 Vacuolated nucleated bone marrow cells in alcoholism. Seminars in Hematology 17: 100

Sullivan L W, Herbert V 1964 Suppression of hematopoiesis by ethanol. Journal of Clinical Investigation 43: 2048

Question 61

Ansell B M 1970 Henoch-Schönlein purpura with particular reference to the prognosis of the renal lesion. British Journal of Dermatology 82: 211

Kreidberg M B, Dameshek W, Latoracca R 1955 Acute vascular purpura (Schönlein-Henoch): an immunological disease. New England Journal of Medicine 253: 1014

Levinsky R J, Barratt T M 1979 IgA immune complexes in Henoch-Schonlein purpura. Lancet ii: 1100

Question 62

Cohen A S 1967 Amyloidosis. New England Journal of Medicine 277: 522, 574, 628

Isobe T, Osserman E 1974 Patterns of amyloidosis and their association with plasma cell dyscrasias, monoclonal immunoglobulins and Bence-Jones proteins. New England Journal of Medicine 290: 473

Question 63
Frangione B, Franklin E C 1973 Heavy chain diseases: clinical features and molecular significance of the disordered immunoglobulin structure. Seminars in Hematology 10: 53
Questions 64 & 65
Fessas P, Loukopoulos D 1974 The beta thalassaemias. Clinics in Haematology 3: 411
Wasi P, Na-Nakorn S, Pootrakul S 1974 The alpha thalassaemias. Clinics in Haematology 3: 383
Weatherall D J, Clegg J B 1981 The thalassaemia syndromes, 3rd edn. Blackwell Scientific Publications, Oxford
Questions 66, 67, 68, 69
Bollum F J 1979 Terminal deoxynucleotidyl transferase as a hemopoietic cell marker. Blood 54: 1203
Foucar K, Rydell R E 1980 Richter's syndrome in chronic lymphocytic leukaemia. Cancer 46: 118
Goldman J M, Preisler H D (eds) 1984 Leukaemias. In: International medical reviews: Haematology 1. Butterworths, London
Hart J S, Trujillo J M, Freireich E J, George S L, Frei E III 1971 Cytogenetic studies and their clinical correlation in adults with acute leukaemia. Annals of Internal Medicine 75: 353
Jacqillat L I, Weil M, Geman M F et al 1973 Evaluation of 216 four-year survivors of acute leukaemia. Cancer 32: 286
Robinson L L, Nesbit M E, Sather H N, Hammond G D, Coccia P F 1980 Assessment of the interrelationship of prognostic factors in childhood acute lymphoblastic leukaemia: A report from Children's Cancer Study Group. American Journal of Pediatric Hematology and Oncology 2: 5
Steinhertz P G 1987 Acute lymphoblastic leukaemia of childhood. In: Hematology/Oncology Clinics of North America 1(4): 549
Question 70
Callender S T (ed) 1973 Iron deficiency and iron overload. Clinics in Haematology 2(2): 241
England J M, Fraser P M 1973 Differentiation of iron deficiency from thalassaemia trait by routine blood count. Lancet i: 449
Kasper C K, Whissel D Y E, Wallerstein R O 1965 Clinical aspects of iron deficiency. Journal of the American Medical Association 191: 359
Question 71
Lawler S D 1984 Leucocyte and platelet antigens and antibodies. In: Dacie J V, Lewis S M (eds) Practical haematology, 6th edn Churchill Livingstone, Edinburgh, p 407
Question 72
Dinol K, Aksoy M 1969 On the platelet levels in chronic iron deficiency anaemia. Acta Haematologica 41: 135
Marchasin S, Wallerstein R O 1964 The treatment of iron-deficiency anaemia with intravenous iron dextran. Blood 23: 345
Question 73
Galton D A G, Goldman J M, Wiltshaw E, Catovsky D, Henry K, Goldenberg J 1974 Prolymphocytic leukaemia. British Journal of Haematology 27: 7
Question 74
Hansen N E, Killman S A 1968 Paroxysmal nocturnal haemoglobinuria. A clinical study. Acta Medica Scandinavica 184: 525
Lipson R L, Bayrd E D, Watkins C H 1959 The postsplenectomy blood picture. American Journal of Clinical Pathology 32: 526

Richardson J S, Sarkany I, Cambell C D 1964 Fatal case of marrow aplasia after treatment with carbimazole. British Medical Journal 1: 364
Question 75
Moller G 1973 T and B lymphocytes. Transplant Reviews 16: 3
Warner N L 1974 Membrane immunoglobulins and antigen receptors and T and B lymphocytes. Advances in Immunology 19: 67
Question 76
Schlichter S J, Harker L A 1976 Preparation and storage of platelet concentrates. British Journal of Haematology 34: 403
Sprague C C, Harrington W J, Lange R D, Shapleigh J B 1952 Platelet transfusion and the pathogenesis of idiopathic thrombocytopenic purpura. Journal of the American Medical Association 150: 1193
Question 77
Hardy W R, Anderson R E 1968 The hypereosinophilic syndromes. Annals of Internal Medicine 68: 1120
Major R M, Leget L H 1939 Marked eosinophilia in Hodgkin's disease. Journal of the American Medical Association 112: 2601
Question 78
Burkitt D P, O'Connor G T 1961 Malignant lymphoma in African children, 1. A clinical syndrome. Cancer 14: 258
Mann R B, Berard C W 1977 Burkitt's tumour: lessons from mice, monkeys, and man. Lancet ii: 84
Question 79
Moller G 1973 T and B lymphocytes. Transplant Reviews 16: 3
Question 80
Quinnan G V Jr 1986 Inactivation of HTLV III virus by heat, chemicals and irradiation. Transfusion 26(5): 481
Scully C et al 1986 Acquired immune deficiency syndrome: review. British Dental Journal 161(2): 53
Question 81
Ishizaka K, Ishizaka T 1970 Biologic function of IgE antibodies and mechanisms of reaginic hypersensitivity. Clinical and Experimental Immunology 6: 25
Lennox E S, Cohn M 1967 Immunoglobulins. Annual Review of Biochemistry 36: 365
Merler E, Rosen F S 1966 The gamma globulins. I. Structure and synthesis of the immunoglobulins. New England Journal of Medicine 275: 480
Question 82
Jaffe E S, Blattner W A, Blayney D W et al 1984 The pathologic spectrum of adult T-cell leukaemia/lymphoma in the United States: human T-cell leukaemia/lymphoma virus associated lymphoid malignancies. American Journal of Surgical Pathology 8: 263
Wong-Staal F, Gallo R C 1985 Human T-lymphotropic retroviruses. Nature 317: 395
Question 83
Jones S E 1974 Clinical features and course of the non-Hodgkin's lymphomas. Clinics in Haematology 3(1): 131
Question 84
Forman S J, Farbstein M J, Scott E P et al 1982 Prevention and therapy of graft-versus-host disease. New England Journal of Medicine 307: 376
Glucksberg H, Storb R, Fefer A et al 1974 Clinical manifestations of graft-versus-host disease in human recipients of marrow from HLA-matched sibling donors. Transplantation 18: 295

Question 85
Moran E M, Ultmann J E 1974 Clinical features and course of Hodgkin's disease. Clinics in Haematology 3(1): 91
Question 86
MacKenzie M R, Fundenberg H H 1972 Macroglobulinaemia: an analysis of 40 patients. Blood 39: 874
Question 87
Blume K G et al Bone-marrow ablation and allogeneic marrow transplantation in acute leukaemia. New England Journal of Medicine 302: 1041
Goldman J M, Baughan A S J, McCarthy D M et al 1982 Marrow transplantation for patients in the chronic phase of chronic granulocytic leukaemia. Lancet ii: 623
UCLA Bone Marrow Transplant Team 1976 Bone-marrow transplantation in severe aplastic anaemia. Lancet ii: 921
Question 88
Lutzner M A, Edelson R L, Schein P S, Green I, Kirkpatrick C, Ahmed A T 1975 Cutaneous T-cell lymphoma: the Sezary syndrome, mycosis fungoides, and related disorders. Annals of Internal Medicine 83: 534
Question 89
Goldfinger D, McGuiness M H 1971 Rh-incompatible platelet transfusions — risks and consequences of sensitising immunosuppressed patients. New England Journal of Medicine 284: 942
Pollack W, Ascari W Q, Crispen J F, Oconnor R R, Ho T Y 1971 Studies on Rh prophylaxis II. Rh immune prophylaxis after transfusion with Rh-positive blood. Transfusion 11: 340
Question 90
Cooper R A, Jandl J H 1966 Obstructive jaundice — selective increase in erythrocyte cholesterol in target cells. Clinical Research 14: 314
Question 91
McGarth M A, Penny R 1976 Paraproteinaemia: Blood hyperviscosity and clinical manifestations. Journal of Clinical Investigation 58: 1155

2 MRCP Data Interpretation

Read carefully the clinical and laboratory data provided and answer the questions that follow.

Data Interpretation 1

A 19-year-old Asian woman attended the antenatal clinic. Her blood count showed: WBC 12 $\times$ 10^9/l, RBC 4.44 $\times$ 10^{12}/l, Hgb 9.7 g/dl, PCV .297, MCV 67.0 fl, MCH 21.8 pg, MCHC 32.6 g/dl, RDW 18.3, platelets 396 $\times$ 10^9/l, Pct .295%, MPV 8.4, PDW 16.3. Her diet appears to be satisfactory. On examination she is found to be 24 weeks pregnant.

What further investigations should be performed?

Data Interpretation 2

A 16-year-old boy from Southern India presented with an eight hour history of priapism. His past medical history included attacks of 'rheumatism', and two attacks of malaria, during one of which he developed pneumonia. On examination, he is clinically anaemic and has a very painful engorged penis. There is 4 cm smooth hepatomegaly and a systolic ejection murmur. He is febrile, 39.2°C, and has sinus tachycardia of 115 beats per minute.
Blood count: WBC 27.8 $\times$ 10^9/l, haemoglobin 8.2 g/dl, MCV 80 fl, platelets 510 $\times$ 10^9/l

1. What is the most likely diagnosis?
2. Give three investigations that will confirm the diagnosis.
3. Detail five important aspects of management.

Data Interpretation 3

A 6-year-old boy presents with a painful, swollen right knee. He had previously had several attacks of swelling and pain in the same knee and in view of widespread bruising it was suspected that the child was being mistreated at home. In order to exclude a haemostatic defect a coagulation screen was performed:

Haemoglobin	12.3 g/dl
Platelets	379×10^9/l
Bleeding time (template)	7.5 min
Prothrombin time	14 s (control 12 s)
Thrombin time	13 s (control 12 s)
APTT	59 s (control 33 s)
APTT 50/50 mixture with normal plasma	35 s
Factor VIII:C	0.79 iu/ml
Factor VIII:vWFag	0.83 u/ml

1. Comment on these results.
2. What is the most relevant further laboratory test required to establish a diagnosis?

Data Interpretation 4

The following are results of Schilling tests performed on two patients with megaloblastic anaemia:

	Isotope	*24-hour urine volume*	*% Radioactivity*
Patient 1	[^{57}Co] B_{12}	1700 ml	14%
	[^{57}Co] B_{12} + intrinsic factor	2000 ml	25%
Patient 2	[^{57}] B_{12}	1960 ml	2%
	[^{57}Co] B_{12} + intrinsic factor	1800 ml	6%

What conclusions can you draw about these patients from the results?

Data Interpretation 5

Mrs AS, aged 25 years, visited her GP complaining of heavy menstrual blood loss and fatigue. She had three children, and her periods had been heavy since her last child was born six months previously. On examination there are no abnormalities of note apart from mild pallor. She is Scottish in origin although her family have lived in England all their lives. A blood count revealed a haemoglobin of 8.0 g/dl, PCV 0.36, RBC 6.4 $\times$ 10^{12}/l, MCV 60 fl and platelets 456 $\times$ 10^{9}/l with a normal white count and differential.

1. What is the most likely diagnosis?
2. What further investigations would you carry out?
3. What difficulties may you encounter in reaching a diagnosis?

Data Interpretation 6

A 78-year-old woman is seen in the outpatients department. Three years before she had been diagnosed as having pernicious anaemia on the basis of a macrocytic anaemia, low serum B_{12}, and presence of parietal cell antibodies in the serum. A Schilling test at that time had shown reduced absorption of B_{12}, corrected by addition of intrinsic factor. Since then she had been treated by i.m. hydroxocobalamin 1 mg every third month. Her GP had referred her because of recurrence of her anaemia. Her daughter had noted that she was increasingly depressed and had gained weight.

On examination she was noted to be pale, with vitiligo of both arms. Blood pressure was 120/60, pulse 64/min regular. Auscultation of the heart was normal, but there were bilateral basal crepitations in the chest. Abdominal examination was normal. There was bilateral ankle oedema.

Blood count: WBC 4.8 $\times$ 10^{9}/l, RBC 3.08 $\times$ 10^{12}/l, Hb 9.5 g/dl, PVC .309, MCV 102 fl, MCH 34.1 pg, MCHC 34.0 g/dl, RDW 13.1, platelets 201 $\times$ 10^{9}/l.

1. Is the recurrence of her anaemia likely to be due to inadequate therapy of her pernicious anaemia?
2. Suggest three possible causes for her anaemia.
3. Is the presence of parietal cell antibodies an important criterion for the diagnosis of pernicious anaemia?

Data Interpretation 7

A full blood count sample arrived from Main Theatres. The information given was 'Philips, male, respiratory arrest'.

The blood count and film appearances are as follows: WBC 16.8 × 10^9/l, Hb 19.2 g/dl, PCV 58.2, MCV 104 fl, platelets 387 × 10^9/l. Differential: neutrophils 37%, lymphocytes 57%, monocytes 3%, myelocytes 3%. The blood film showed a few spherocytes, occasional nucleated red cells, a few target cells and macrocytes.

Comment on the haematological findings.

Data Interpretation 8

Mr AJ was aged 48 and had been on medication for hypertension for two years, after his GP noted (on a routine medical examination) that his diastolic blood pressure was 110 mm/Hg. He complained to his GP of a lump in the side of the neck. He was referred to hospital where, on examination, he was found to have bilateral axillary and cervical lymphadenopathy. He was noted to be mildly icteric and short of breath at rest.

A blood count revealed a haemoglobin of 8.0 g, platelets of 265 × 10^9/l and a white count of 14.0 × 10^9/l with 27% neutrophils and 73% mature lymphocytes.

1. Discuss the possible diagnoses.
2. What further tests would you order?

Data Interpretation 9

A 52-year-old woman is admitted as an emergency with a five day history of vomiting and a four week history of polyuria, polydipsia, headache, increasing deafness and constipation. On examination the positive findings are that she is dehydrated, has small areas of bruising and is very tender on palpation of the rib-cage. Fundoscopy showed dilated tortuous veins but no papilloedema.

WBC 3.6 × 10^9/l, haemoglobin 8.5 g/dl, platelets 105 × 10^9/l. Normal differential.

Urea 18.6 mmol/l, creatinine 345 mmol/l, total protein 115 g/l, albumin 29 g/l, blood glucose 6.4 mmol/l.

1. What are the two most important emergency investigations?
2. What single diagnosis would best explain the findings?
3. Give four investigations necessary to establish the diagnosis.

Data Interpretation 10

A 5-year-old boy is seen in the ENT clinic with a history of recurrent tonsillitis. On examination he is found to have enlarged tonsils, but the examining surgeon is alarmed to note that he is centrally cyanosed. Following referral to a physician the child's blood is found to contain 20% methaemoglobin.

Which of the following facts in the history may be relevant?

1. His farming family draw their drinking water from a well.
2. He had received a course of erythromycin from his GP the previous week.
3. He is very fond of German sausage.
4. There is a strong paternal history of ischaemic heart disease.
5. He helps his sister tie-dye T-shirts for her market stall.

Data Interpretation 11

A 69-year-old man has the following blood count: WBC 6.1 $\times 10^9$/l, RBC 2.47 $\times 10^{12}$/l, Hb 7.6 g/dl, PCV .231, MCV 93.5 fl, MCH 30.8 pg, MCHC 32.9 g/dl, platelets 341 $\times 10^9$/l. Differential: neutrophils 39%, lymphocytes 52%, monocytes 5%, eosinophils 1%, metamyelocytes 2%, myelocytes 1%. 3 nucleated RBC/100 WBC.

Which of the following investigations are indicated and why?

1. Serum iron and total iron binding capacity.
2. Red cell mass/plasma volume estimation.
3. Serum acid phosphate.
4. Bone marrow biopsy.
5. Serum protein electrophoresis.

Data Interpretation 12

Mr AH, aged 53, worked as an advertising executive, and a routine blood test showed him to have a haemoglobin of 19.4 g/dl with a normal platelet and white count. His PCV is .55. He smokes heavily but chest X-ray is normal. On examination he is obese and rather plethoric. There are no other physical abnormalities.

What are the possible diagnoses, and how would you investigate this man?

Data Interpretation 13

	Patient's serum with:				Patient's cells with:		
	Own cells	*A cells*	*B cells*	*O cells*	*Anti-A*	*Anti-B*	*Anti-A,B*
1.	−	++	++	−	−	−	−
2.	+++	+++	+++	+++	++	−	++
3.	−	−	−	−	−	−	−
4.	−	++	++	++	−	++	++
5.	−	−	++	−	++	−	++

Interpret the blood group findings shown above.

Data Interpretation 14

An 18-year-old black soldier attends morning sick-parade complaining of passing 'coca-cola' urine and muscular aches and pains. He had completed a 20 mile march the day before.

Physical examination showed no abnormalities. Urine microscopy showed no red cells or white cells, though a 'Haemastik' test gave positive results.

1. Suggest three possible diagnoses.
2. What further investigations would be necessary to confirm them?

Data Interpretation 15

A 20-year-old Caucasian woman attended the antenatal clinic for booking in her first pregnancy. A palpable spleen was found on abdominal examination. There was no significant family or drug history, but she had had two episodes of jaundice in childhood.

Blood count: WBC 12.5 × 10^9/l, RBC 2.7 × 10^{12}/l, Hb 9.3 g/dl, PCV .257, MCV 96.1 fl, MCH 32.4 pg, MCHC 36.2 g/dl, RDW 21.2, platelets 438 × 10^9/l

Differential: neutrophils 71%, lymphocytes 26%, monocytes 3%. Film: polychromasia and spherocytes present. Reticulocyte count 12%. Blood group: A Rh negative. Screen for atypical red cell antibodies: negative. Direct antiglobulin test: negative.

1. What diagnosis do you suspect?
2. What confirmatory investigation should be performed?
3. What treatment should she have during pregnancy?

Data Interpretation 16

A 58-year-old Caucasian man visited his general practitioner complaining of feeling 'off colour'. His wife had died a year before. He denied shortness of breath or weight loss, but had a poor appetite. He had been taking ibuprofen for backache for two years.

On physical examination pallor was the only abnormality.

Blood count: WBC 4.9 × 10^9/l, RBC 4.43 × 10^{12}/l, Hb 9.6 g/dl, PCV 30.1, MCV 67.9 fl, MCH 21.7 pg, MCHC 31.9 g/l, RDW 19.9, platelets 515 × 10^9/l. Differential: neutrophils 60%, lymphocytes 33%, monocytes 7%. ESR 65 mm/h

1. What is the most likely cause of his anaemia, and how may you confirm it?
2. What further points would you wish to elicit in the history?
3. What further investigations would you wish to perform?

Data Interpretation 17

A 67-year-old widower presented with progressive lethargy and recent swelling of the ankles. For the last few weeks he had been having difficulty with walking, and angina of effort. On examination he was very pale, had mild bilateral heart failure, and his spleen tip was palpable. Examination of the cranial nerves was normal, but there was loss of vibration and position sense in the lower legs. The knee and ankle jerks were absent bilaterally, and the plantar responses were extensor.

Blood count: WBC 1.9 × 10^9/l, Hb 2.8 g/dl, MCV 122 fl, platelets 95 × 10^9/l.

1. What is the most likely diagnosis?
2. What is the differential diagnosis of the neurological signs?
3. How would you manage this patient?

Data Interpretation 18

A 24-year-old Italian woman living in the UK returned to Rome to visit her parents for one week. One week later she felt unwell with fever, vague headaches and lower abdominal discomfort. She was thought to have a urinary tract infection.

Blood cultures were taken, and she was started on ampicillin as an outpatient. A full blood count at this time was normal. Over the next few days she became progressively unwell with severe headaches, a high swinging fever and rigors. On admission to hospital her temperture was 39.6°C, she was hypotensive, semi-comatose and there was a suggestion of peritonism. Her urine was noted to be black and found to contain free haemoglobin. The blood cultures taken three days before were sterile.

Blood count: WBC 10.4 × 10^9/l, Hb 8.7 g/dl, MCV 96 fl, platelets 40 × 10^9/l. Differential: neutrophils 82%, lymphocytes 14%, monocytes 4%. Blood film: shows polychromasia and microangiopathic changes. Reticulocyte count 5%. Sickle test:negative.

1. State two possible diagnoses.
2. What three investigations would you perform next?

Data Interpretation 19

Mr DS aged 21, presented with gum bleeding and nose bleeds. Examination revealed widespread purpura and pallor of mucous membranes. There was little of significance in his past medical history except for an episode of jaundice and vomiting following a holiday in Southern Italy, one year before.

Blood count: WBC 1.9×10^9/l, haemoglobin 7.5 g/dl, MCV 101 fl, platelets 27×10^9/l. Differential: neutrophils 10%, lymphocytes 88%, monocytes 2%.

1. What are the two most likely diagnoses?
2. What is the most important investigation that you would carry out?

Data Interpretation 20

A 25-year-old woman was admitted in labour with a 36-week gestation and a two week history of jaundice. Within hours she delivered viable twins but uterine atony and persistent vaginal haemorrhage, (estimated to be 1500 ml) followed, associated with excessive bleeding from venepuncture sites. She was transfused with compatible packed red cells, and a coagulation screen obtained:

Haemoglobin	7.9 g/dl
Platelets	49×10^9/l
Prothrombin time	17 s (control 14 s)
APTT	51 s (control 33 s)
APTT	50/50 mix with normal plasma 37 s
Thrombin time	38 s (control 12 s)
Fibrinogen	1.2 g/l
Fibrin degradation products	$> 20 < 40$ μg/ml
Antithrombin III	0.47 iu/ml (normal range 0.8–1.2)

Comment on these results and discuss the future management of this patient.

Data Interpretation 21

A 37-year-old Indian woman complained of tiredness, heavy periods, depression and occasional nose bleeds. On examination she has a spleen palpable to the umbilicus and a three cm palpable liver. She stated that her spleen has been palpable since early childhood in India.

Blood count: WBC 1.3 × 10^9/l, Hb 4.4 g/dl, MCV 57 fl, MCH 16.2 pg, platelets 121 × 10^9/l. Differential: normal. Reticulocyte count 5%.

1. Comment on the haematological results in relation to the clinical presentation.
2. What three investigations would most help in confirming the haematological diagnosis?
3. Suggest two likely causes for the splenomegaly.

Data Interpretation 22

A 63-year-old woman was admitted with a suspected diagnosis of obstructive jaundice secondary to carcinoma of the pancreas. Prior to an ERCP procedure a coagulation screen was performed:

Haemoglobin	11.7 g/dl
Platelets	157 × 10^9/l
Bleeding time (template method)	8 min
Prothrombin time	34 s (control 13 s)
Thrombin time	21 s (control 13 s)
APTT	41 s (control 35 s)
APTT 50/50 mix with normal plasma	37 s
Factor V assay	0.41 u/ml
Factor X assay	0.34 u/ml

Comment on these results and discuss what specific therapy should be undertaken to prevent bleeding complications prior to the ERCP.

Data Interpretation 23

A 22-year-old Indian woman, para 1, is seen at the booking antenatal clinic. She is a strict vegetarian. Her blood count at this time is as follows: WBC 10.7 × 10^9/l, Hb 13.0 g/dl, MCV

86 fl, platelets 260 × 10^9/l. At 36 weeks gestation she is noted to have WBC 11.0 × 10^9/l, Hb 9.1 g/dl, MCV 108, platelets 260 × 10^9/l. She is empirically given supplements of iron and folic acid, but in retrospect serum iron and folate levels at this stage were normal.

At term her blood count shows WBC 3.3 × 10^9/l, Hb 8.5 g/dl, MCV 108 fl, platelets 110 × 10^9/l. Reticulocyte count is 1.5%. Hypersegmented neutrophils are seen in the film.

1. What is the likely cause of her anaemia?
2. Is this common in pregnancy?

Data Interpretation 24

A 45-year-old man is admitted following a large haematemesis. He has signs of hypovolaemic shock, and an immediate transfusion of 'emergency' group O Rh negative blood is given. Fully cross-matched blood is later available and he receives a total of six units. A similar episode occurred two years previously.

Four days after admission he is visibly jaundiced but otherwise well. His liver function tests show: bilirubin 40 μmol/l, aspartate aminotransferase and alkaline phosphatase normal, direct antiglobulin test positive (mixed field reaction), Schumm's test negative, serum haptoglobins absent, renal function normal. Patient's blood group: A Rh positive (genotype R_1R_1, CDe/CDe). Patient's serum contains anti-c and anti-E.

1. Has the patient received incompatible blood? State your reasoning.
2. Is it likely from the patient's clinical state and results that he has suffered a significant haemolytic transfusion reaction?

Data Interpretation 25

An elderly vagrant was admitted with acute bronchopneumonia. No further history was available.

A blood count was as follows: WBC 3.5 × 10^9/l, Hb 7.9 g/dl, MCV 105 fl, platelets 105 × 10^9/l. Neutrophils 2.4 × 10^9/l. A blood film showed spur cells and occasional stomatocytes. Bone marrow aspirate showed moderate hypocellularity with a myeloid:erythroid ration of 2.4:1. Erythropoiesis was dysplastic with vacuolated normoblasts. Iron stain showed numerous ringed sideroblasts.

1. What is the single most likely cause of the haematological abnormalities?
2. It is later learnt that the patient has been receiving therapy for tuberculosis for the previous seven months. How might this have influenced the haematological findings?

Data Interpretation 26

A 34-year-old woman attended the gynaecology clinic for longstanding menorrhagia. She had felt lethargic for many months and had taken a succession of vitamin preparations and herbal remedies without improvement. A blood count was as follows:
WBC 7.1 $\times$ 10^9/l, Hb 9.1 g/dl, MCV 80 fl, platelets 380 $\times$ 10^9/l. Differential: neutrophils 59%, lymphocytes 59%, monocytes 5%. Blood film: a dimorphic picture with some normal red cells and some microcytic hypochromic cells.

1. What is the likely diagnosis?
2. How would you confirm the diagnosis?

Answers/Comments

Data Interpretation Answer 1

This patient has a microcytic hypochromic anaemia, and measurement of serum iron and TIBC may provide a guide to her iron status. However, the serum iron may be falsely elevated if estimated when the patient is actually on iron, and the TIBC is elevated in the third trimester even in women who are not iron deficient.

The haemoglobin A_2 level should be estimated as β-thalassaemia trait has an incidence of 3–10% in Asian patients. This causes a microcytic/hypochromic picture mimicking iron deficiency, with an elevated haemoglobin A_2 level. A neutrophilia is normal in pregnancy.

Data Interpretation Answer 2

The most likely diagnosis is vaso-occlusive crisis (of the penis) due to sickle cell disease (SCD). There is a high gene frequency for HbS in Southern India. A leukaemia, e.g. CGL, is possible but priapism secondary to blood hyperviscosity would not be seen at such a comparatively low white cell count. All the other clinical features are consistent with SCD. The hyposplenism seen in adults with SCD will explain the neutrophilia and thrombocytosis, but both may be more marked during vaso-occlusive crisis.

The diagnosis may be confirmed by examination of the blood film, sickle solubility test and haemoglobin electrophoresis. Important aspects of management include adequate analgesia and liaison with genitourinary surgeons in case a definitive surgical procedure is necessary. Underlying infection should be sought and treated if present. 'Blind' wide-spectrum antibiotics, e.g. amoxycillin, are often given in vaso-occlusive crisis but their benefit is unproven. Adequate hydration is important.

Oxygen therapy is not usually helpful in local vaso-occlusion but, at levels below 35% inspired air, it can do no harm. Bed rest and warmth are important. If SCD is newly diagnosed the family will need counselling. Exchange blood transfusion may be necessary if the priapism does not resolve within twelve hours or so, but its use is controversial.

Data Interpretation Answer 3

The coagulation screen shows a prolonged APTT, which fully corrects when the patient's plasma is incubated with 50% normal plasma, with a normal prothrombin and thrombin time. This suggests a deficiency of factor VIII, IX, XI, XII or one of the contact factors, (HMW kininogen or prekallikrein). In a 6-year-old boy this is most likely to be a congential deficiency of factor VIII:C, (classical haemophilia A). However, factor VIII:C and VIII:vWFag assays were both within the normal range of 0.5–2.0 iu/ml, (equivalent to 50–200%), which excludes a diagnosis of haemophilia A. The other possible factor deficiencies should then be excluded. Of these factor IX deficiency, (Christmas disease or haemophilia B), is the most likely, and moderate to severe deficiency may cause spontaneous haemarthroses and easy bruising. A factor IX:C assay of 0.14 u/ml subsequently confirmed a diagnosis of Christmas disease.

Data Interpretation Answer 4

All the urine collections appear to be of adequate volume. In Patient 1 both results are well within the normal range, whereas in Patient 2, both results are subnormal ($<$ 10% excretion).

The addition of intrinsic factor (IF) often leads to some increase in excretion even when lack of IF is not the cause of B_{12} deficiency, and hence the higher results with IF in both patients. Once a normal result is obtained in a part I Schilling, it is not necessary to proceed to part II. The megaloblastic anaemia in Patient 1 is therefore due to dietary B_{12} deficiency (or some other cause, e.g. folate deficiency, which should have been excluded before proceeding to a Schilling test). Patient 2 may have disease of the terminal ileum preventing absorption of B_{12} even with intrinsic factor.

Data Interpretation Answer 5

Menorrhagia suggests a diagnosis of iron deficiency, although clinical enquiry alone makes it hard to establish the extent of the problem. The high red cell count with the low MCV raises the possibility of β-thalassaemia trait. The slightly raised platelet count and the haemoglobin of 8.0 g/dl (unusually low for β-thalassaemia trait) suggests a diagnosis of iron deficiency. Target cells and hypochromic microcytes are seen in both β-thalassaemia trait and iron deficiency. The presence of pencil cells favours iron deficiency; basophilic stippling favours β-thalassaemia trait. β-thalassaemia trait is classically found in people of Mediterranean origin; however it may be seen in North Europeans. A serum ferritin and iron and iron binding capacity should be requested, and haemoglobin A_2 level measured. A raised A_2 level is found in β-thalassaemia trait. In iron deficiency, the A_2 level may be normal or low even in the presence of β-thalassaemia trait. This woman proved to have iron deficiency in addition to β-thalassaemia trait. Iron therapy and a dilatation and curettage improved the former problem, a haemoglobin of 11.0 g/dl resulting. Initially her A_2 level was normal, but following therapy with oral iron this rose to 4.1%.

Data Interpretation Answer 6

The WHO recommendation for vitamin B_{12} maintenance treatment in pernicious anaemia is hydroxocobalamin 1 mg every third month. Hydroxocobalamin is better retained in the body than cyanocobalamin and may be more effective in the correction of the optic complications of B_{12} deficiency. Cyanocobalamin is still used in the Schilling test however.

Possible causes of her anaemia are hypothyroidism, folic acid deficiency and bleeding (e.g. from carcinoma of the stomach).

Many elderly people have parietal cell antibodies. The presence of intrinsic factor antibodies is more significant and specific. However the diagnosis of pernicious anaemia still rests on the demonstration of impaired B_{12} absorption in the part I Schilling test, corrected by the addition of intrinsic factor in the part II Schilling test.

On investigation this woman was found to be hypothyroid with positive thyroid auto-antibodies.

Data Interpretation Answer 7

Macrocytosis, polycythaemia, lymphocytosis and leucoerythroblastic film are all normal findings in a neonate.

Data Interpretation Answer 8

His blood count and physical examination suggest a lymphoproliferative disorder, so marker studies i.e. cellular antigen studies, should be carried out on the lymphoid cells. A bone marrow examination with a trephine may be helpful. Anaemia with jaundice suggests haemolysis. He has been on medication for hypertension so it should be ascertained whether this was methyldopa, known to cause autoimmune haemolytic anaemia in approximately 1% of patients. An unconjugated bilirubin estimation, and direct antiglobulin test should be performed, also the reticulocyte count and serum haptoglobin level.

This patient had a positive direct antiglobulin test and anti-e was detected on his red cells after antibody elution. This is the antibody most commonly associated with methyldopa therapy. Methyldopa was discontinued for six months but his direct antiglobulin test remained positive although the haemolysis ceased.

A diagnosis of chronic lymphocytic leukaemia was made on his bone marrow and markers. Chronic lymphocytic leukaemia may be associated with haemolytic anaemia, most commonly due to a warm antibody.

Data Interpretation Answer 9

This middle-aged woman has bony tenderness and the classical features of hypercalcaemia (polyuria, thirst, anorexia, vomiting, constipation and muscle fatigue) and hyperviscosity syndrome (visual disturbance, weakness, headache, hearing loss, convulsions, bleeding diathesis and cardiac failure). She is anaemic and thrombocytopenic, has renal impairment and a very high serum protein. The most likely diagnosis is myeloma. Hypercalcaemia and hyperviscosity are both potentially fatal but amenable to emergency treatment. The serum calcium and plasma viscosity should be measured urgently. Diagnostic investigations for myeloma should include serum protein electrophoresis, bone marrow aspirate, further studies to qualify and quantify the the monoclonal paraprotein and full radiological skeletal survey to look for lytic lesions and pathological fractures (isotope bone scans are not helpful in myeloma except to confirm fracture sites). An early morning urine should be collected to look for Bence-Jones proteinuria (free light chains). The ESR is often very high in myeloma but it is a non-specific test.

Data Interpretation Answer 10

Methaemoglobin is oxidised haemoglobin. Normally the enzyme methaemoglobin reductase is responsible for the reconversion of methaemoglobin to haemoglobin. Congenital deficiency of methaemoglobin reductase may result in methaemoglobinaemia. Also, exposure of some individuals to various oxidant drugs and chemicals may result in methaemoglobinaemia. Contamination of drinking water by nitrate fertilisers may be a cause. Erythromycin does not cause methaemoglobinaemia, however some sulphonamides have been implicated. Nitrate is used as a meat preservative, and may cause methaemoglobinaemia in susceptible individuals. Aniline dyes, some of which may be absorbed through the skin, may cause methaemoglobinaemia.

Data Interpretation Answer 11

The blood count shows a *leucoerythroblastic picture*, that is the presence of nucleated red cells and primitive white cells of any variety in the peripheral blood, usually with anaemia. Unless the patient is critically ill (major trauma, septicaemia etc.) it is an indication of bone marrow infiltration. The anaemia is normocytic and normochromic, not suggestive of iron deficiency. The haemoglobin level demonstrates a low red cell mass and red cell mass estimation is not indicated. Carcinoma of the prostate infiltrating marrow is a possible diagnosis, and a raised acid phosphatase may provide a marker for this disease. Carcinomas that commonly spread to bone include prostate, breast, lung, thyroid, kidney. To demonstrate marrow infiltration by carcinoma, lymphoma, myelofibrosis or myeloma, bone marrow biopsy is indicated. A serum paraprotein is present in myeloma.

Data Interpretation Answer 12

This man either has primary polycythaemia — polycythaemia rubra vera — or secondary polycythaemia, perhaps secondary to smoking. Finally he could have 'stress polycythaemia' or pseudopolycythaemia, so-called Gaisboeck syndrome.

A red cell mass and plasma volume estimation was performed, which showed a red cell mass of 31 ml/kg (normal for males 25–35 ml/kg) and a plasma volume of 35 ml/kg (normal 40–50 ml/kg). Other initial investigations included blood gases, which showed a pO_2 of 98 mmHg with a normal CO_2.

The reduced plasma volume is in keeping with a diagnosis of pseudopolycythaemia. Had the red cell mass been raised then appropriate investigations would have included neutrophil alkaline phosphatase (NAP) score, raised in polycythaemia rubra vera (PRV), and bone marrow biopsy to look for fibrosis associated with PRV. Renal causes of polycythaemia should be excluded by an examination of a urinary deposit and abdominal ultrasound. The latter may also assess spleen size, splenomegaly being common in PRV.

This patient was advised to stop smoking, lose weight and take a holiday. Six months later his haemoglobin was 17.5 g/dl with a PCV of .51.

Data Interpretation Answer 13

(Refer to table on p. 80.)

1. Normal group O. The serum contains naturally occurring anti-A and anti-B; the cells do not group with antisera to group A or B.
2. Group A but with auto-immune red cell antibodies. The patient's serum reacts with his own red cells. It is impossible to say without further investigation against which red cell antigen the auto-antibody is directed, therefore the serum grouping (which appears to be against A, B and O cells) is uninterpretable. The cell grouping however is group A.
3. Group O with apparently no 'naturally occurring' anti-A or

anti-B. This occurs in the normal neonate and also in rare adults who are severely hypogammaglobinaemic.

4. Group B with atypical red cell allo-antibodies. The cell group is clearly B but the patient's serum appears to react not only against the expected A cells, but also against B cells and O cells. There is no reaction with their own cells. The explanation would be that the patient's serum contains an antibody that is reacting, not against the B antigen or the 'O' antigen but against another red cell antigen that, by coincidence, these two test cells carry, e.g. M, N, etc.
5. Normal group A.

Data Interpretation Answer 14

Possible diagnoses in this case include march haemoglobinuria, myoglobinuria, haemoglobinuria associated with sickle cell disease or glucose-6-phosphate dehydrogenase (G6PD) deficiency and paroxysmal cold haemoglobinuria.

The measurement of haemoglobin, MCV, RDW, reticulocyte count, and blood film examination may reveal evidence of haemolysis. Differentiation between haemoglobin and myoglobin in urine can be made in the laboratory as the former is insoluble in ammonium sulphate solution.

Sickle cell haemoglobin screening by electrophoresis or solubility testing is performed on all non-Caucasian military recruits, and sickle cell disease (HbSS, HbSC, Sβ Thal.) sufferers would normally be debarred from military service. Very rarely persons with sickle cell trait may suffer from vaso-occlusive crises during periods of severe physical stress or anoxia.

Haemolysis due to G6PD deficiency will normally be associated with a history of drug ingestion (e.g. anti-malarials) or consumption of fava beans. A G6PD screening test can be performed on the blood.

Paroxysmal cold haemoglobinuria will often be associated with a history of chilling or viral infection and may be confirmed by a positive Donath-Landsteiner test. In this test the patient's blood is incubated at 0°C to allow the cold-acting complement-fixing antibody to fix to the cells, and then warmed to 37°C to allow complement to lyse the cells. (Paroxysmal nocturnal haemoglobinuria almost never presents with visible haemoglobinuria.)

The blood count and film in this case were normal. Sickle solubility test was negative and G6PD screen normal. Further examination of the urine demonstrated haemoglobin. The Donath-Landsteiner test was negative. A diagnosis of march haemoglobinuria was made in this case.

Data Interpretation Answer 15

The most likely diagnosis is hereditary spherocytosis (HS).

An osmotic fragility curve should be performed. The spherocytes found in this condition cannot resist osmotic stress and tend to lyse at higher concentrations of saline than normal (see Fig. 2.1).

In most chronic haemolytic conditions, including HS, treatment with folate supplements is indicated. This is especially important during pregnancy because of the additional folate demand. The usual antenatal combined

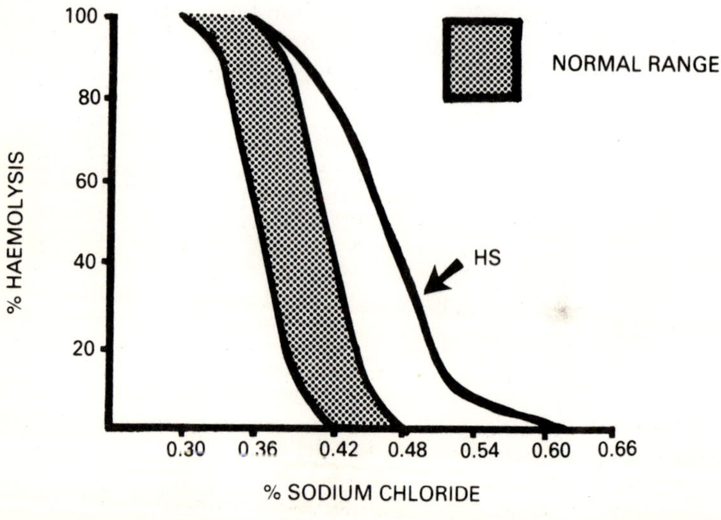

Fig. 2.1 Red cell osmotic fragility curve. The normal range is shaded in and the curve from a patient with hereditary spherocytosis (HS) is shown. The 'tail' of osmotically fragile cells is characteristic.

iron and folate tablets do not provide enough additional folic acid for these patients. This woman may require blood transfusion, particularly if the haemoglobin is still below 10 g/dl close to delivery.

Splenectomy should not be performed during pregnancy because of the risk to the fetus. If anaemia persists after pregnancy, splenectomy will usually restore the haemoglobin to normal levels. Cholecystectomy may be performed at the same time if pigment gallstones have formed.

Approximately three-quarters of cases of HS are autosomal dominantly inherited. However a quarter of all cases, as here, have no family history.

Data Interpretation Answer 16

This is a microcytic hypochromic anaemia most likely due to iron deficiency. Thalassaemia trait should also be considered. The diagnosis may be confirmed by measurement of serum iron (low) and total iron binding capacity (high), measurement of serum ferritin (low), or bone marrow aspirate to assess stainable iron (seldom necessary).

In the history enquiry should be made about any blood loss, particularly melaena, or symptoms of indigestion or abdominal pain. A dietary history should be taken. Without a clear history of blood loss or dietary deficiency chronic gastrointestinal bleeding should be suspected as a cause. Hence occult blood testing, barium meal and enema are appropriate investigations. Non-steroidal anti-inflammatory drug therapy (e.g. ibuprofen) may cause GIT irritation and exacerbate blood loss by impairment of platelet function. The ESR is raised, which is not compatible with simple drug-induced gastritis. On investigation the patient was found to have a colonic carcinoma, which was successfully resected.

Data Interpretation Answer 17

The combination of a severe macrocytic anaemia with pancytopenia and upper and lower motor neurone defects, as well as sensory abnormalities, indicates that the patient is almost certainly suffering from B_{12} deficiency with sub-acute combined degeneration of the cord. The heart failure and angina are largely attributable to the anaemia.

The neurological signs could be due to syphilis although extensor plantars are rare and normal pupils unusual. The combination of upper and lower motor neurone lesions is also seen in motor neurone disease, but the sensory loss is not compatible with this diagnosis. The signs are compatible with Friedreich's ataxia but the age of presentation militates against this.

Appropriate blood samples should be taken to confirm the vitamin B_{12} deficiency and treatment with intramuscular hydroxocobalamin (1 mg) instituted immediately. In view of the severity of the anaemia and the cardiac decompensation, exchange transfusion to raise the haemoglobin slowly without volume overload is indicated. The plasma potassium level should be monitored closely, and potassium supplements given as necessary — hypokalaemia may be severe in the early stages of replacement therapy in severe B_{12} deficiency.

Data Interpretation Answer 18

The history and clinical findings are compatible with a ruptured internal viscus, septicaemia and disseminated intravascular coagulation, even though the original blood cultures were negative. An alternative diagnosis is that of thrombotic thrombocytopenic purpura precipitated by infection. Thirdly, the combination of high swinging fevers, mental confusion, haemolytic anaemia with black urine and thrombocytopenia must raise the possibility of malaria although 'black-water fever' is unusual in previously unaffected individuals.

A thick blood film should be examined immediately for malarial parasites. A full clotting screen should be performed to help discriminate between the above diagnoses (the clotting screen being relatively normal in TTP), and an exploratory laparotomy might be necessary. Blood cultures should be repeated.

Examination of the thick film in this patient revealed *Plasmodium falciparum*. Although malaria is not endemic in

Rome the patient had flown from Rome to London on a flight originating in East Africa. She had so-called 'airport malaria'. Therapy was instituted with intravenous quinine and the outcome was satisfactory.

Data Interpretation Answer 19

Pancytopenia of this order suggests either acute leukaemia or aplastic anaemia. The episode of jaundice raises the possibility of aplasia following hepatitis A. A pancytopenia may be seen in severe megaloblastic anaemia, but it is very rarely this severe and the MCV in this case is only minimally raised. PNH should be excluded with a Ham's test.

A bone marrow aspirate and trephine should be carried out in the first instance to establish the diagnosis.

Other laboratory features of aplastic anaemia are a slight macrocytosis with a low reticulocyte count. Absence of blast cells in the peripheral blood film together with the history of probable hepatitis makes aplastic anaemia the most likely diagnosis. The virus is not only toxic to hepatocytes, but also to the bone marrow stem cells of some individuals. The patient was treated with high-dose methylprednisolone, with some improvement to his blood count, followed by anti-lymphocyte globulin with marked improvement. However this was not sustained, and six months later he received an bone marrow transplant from his monozygotic twin.

Data Interpretation Answer 20

This patient has a prolonged thrombin time and APTT which is associated with mild thrombocytopenia, a low fibrinogen level and slightly raised FDPs (normal $< 20\ \mu g/ml$). These features are diagnostic of acute disseminated intravascular coagulation. This could have been triggered by retained products of conception or acute fatty liver of pregnancy. Immediate haematological treatment must consist of maintaining blood volume and a haematocrit of above 0.30. The haemostatic defects should be controlled so as to control the bleeding and allow safer obstetric management of the precipitating cause. Platelet concentrate, fresh frozen plasma and cryoprecipitate should be transfused and antithrombin III concentrate given (if available). Following infusion of these materials a repeat coagulation screen should be obtained to assess improvement and guide further therapy.

Data Interpretation Answer 21

The patient has a severe and longstanding iron deficiency anaemia, and also a pancytopenia secondary to hypersplenism. The iron deficiency was due to a combination of menorrhagia and poor diet, but gastrointestinal blood loss as well as the nose bleeds may have contributed. The two most useful further investigations would be serum iron and iron binding capacity, to confirm iron deficiency, and bone marrow examination to confirm hypersplenism. Haemoglobin electrophoresis will help to exclude haemoglobin H disease and β-thalassaemia intermedia. The splenomegaly is very longstanding and a malignant cause is unlikely. This patient actually had portal hypertension from congenital hepatic fibrosis, but tropical splenomegaly (secondary to malaria or other tropical causes) and storage diseases such as Gaucher's disease are possible diagnoses.

Data Interpretation Answer 22

This patient has a prolonged APTT, prothrombin time, and thrombin time. The most usual cause of a prolonged APTT and prothrombin time associated with obstructive jaundice is vitamin K deficiency. This causes reduced levels of the vitamin K dependent clotting factors II, VII, IX, and X. This is confirmed by a reduced factor X assay of 0.34 u/ml (normal range 0.5–2.0). However there is always the possibility in this type of patient of direct liver cell damage associated with metastatic carcinoma also contributing to the haemostatic disorder.

Liver damage is suggested by the reduced level of factor V activity, which is not dependent on vitamin K availability, and the prolonged thrombin time. Particularly in metastatic disease, hypofibrinogenaemia and the production of an acquired abnormal fibrinogen molecule may cause a prolonged thrombin time and predispose towards excessive clinical bleeding episodes.

10 mg of vitamin K should be given by slow intravenous injection and the prothrombin time checked after 24 hours. If only partial correction has occurred, an infusion of 2–4 units of fresh frozen plasma should then be given before the ERCP is undertaken.

Data Interpretation Answer 23

The peripheral blood changes are highly suggestive of megaloblastic anaemia, and this was confirmed on bone marrow examination. The serum B_{12} level at 36 weeks was reduced at 129 ng/l, but in a pregnant woman there is a significant fall in serum levels during pregnancy. The level at term was very low (45 ng/l) and the patient's anaemia rapidly responded to vitamin B_{12} supplements. In view of the lack of response to folate, and normal folate levels at 36 weeks, this must be the most likely diagnosis in this case, even though megaloblastic anaemia in pregnancy is very rarely caused by vitamin B_{12} deficiency. Strict vegetarians have a very low B_{12} intake. In retrospect, appropriate therapy of a pregnant woman with an MCV that high would have included 1 mg of i.m. B_{12} while awaiting the results of serum vitamin levels.

Data Interpretation Answer 24

The emergency group O Rh negative (cde/cde) blood contains the antigen c to which the patient has an antibody, which must have been stimulated by his previous blood transfusion. He has therefore received one unit of incompatible blood. Anti-c, unlike ABO haemagglutinins, does not fix complement and produces predominantly extravascular haemolysis. In many cases such haemolytic reactions are suspected because of jaundice a few days after the transfusion, without a great deal of systemic upset. This type of reaction is potentially hazardous and this patient should in an emergency be given group A or group O blood of the genotype R_1R_1 (CDe/CDe).

Data Interpretation Answer 25

The most likely diagnosis is chronic alcoholism. The macrocytic anaemia, with spur cells and stomatocytes, is highly suggestive of this diagnosis. A hypocellular bone marrow is typical and this is reflected by the lack of a neutrophil leucocytosis in response to infection and the mild thrombocytopenia. Vacuolated normoblasts and ringed sideroblasts are common in alcoholism, the latter due to alcohol-induced deficiency of pyridoxal phosphate.

Anti-tuberculous drugs (particularly isoniazid, pyrazinamide, and cycloserine) are a well recognised cause of ringed sideroblasts. Pyrazinamide and isoniazid might also induce hepatic dysfunction which could contribute to the macrocytosis and red cell morphological changes.

Data Interpretation Answer 26

With the history of menorrhagia the most likely cause of the anaemia is iron deficiency. The low normal MCV and the dimorphic blood picture suggest that this has been partially treated. Many proprietary vitamin preparations contain some iron.

The diagnosis should be confirmed by measurement of the serum iron and total iron binding capacity. It should be borne in mind that the serum iron is sometimes misleadingly high in patients taking iron. A serum ferritin level gives a good indication of iron stores in borderline cases. The ultimate diagnostic proof is the haematological response to adequate iron replacement therapy.

FURTHER READING

Question 1

Klee G, Fairbanks V F, Pierre R V, O'Sullivan M B 1976 Use of electronic erythrocyte measurements in the diagnosis of iron deficiency and thalassaemia trait. American Journal of Clinical Pathology 66: 870

Question 2

Charache S 1981 Treatment of sickle cell anaemia. Annual Review of Medicine 32: 195

Question 3

Proctor R R, Rapaport S I 1961 The partial thromboplastin time with kaolin. A simple screening test for first stage plasma clotting factor deficiencies. American Journal of Clinical Pathology 36: 212

Question 4
Akun S N, Miller I F, Meyer L M 1969 Vitamin B_{12} absorption test. Acta Haematologica 41: 341
Question 5
As for MCQ 70, p 71
Question 6
Irvine W J, Davies S H, Delamore J W, Williams A W 1962 Immunologic relationship between pernicious anaemia and thyroid disease. British Medical Journal 2: 454
Larsson S D 1967 Anaemia and iron metabolism in hypothyroidism. Acta Medica Scandinavia 157: 349
Question 7
Schwartz E, Gill F M 1986 Hematology of the newborn. In: Williams W J, Beutler E, Eisler A J, Lichtman M A (eds) Hematology, 3rd edn. McGraw-Hill, New York, p 37
Question 8
Worrlege S M, Carstairs K C, Dacie J V 1966 Autoimmune haemolytic anaemia associated with alpha-methyldopa therapy Lancet ii: 133
Question 9
Salmon S E (ed) 1982 Myeloma and related disorders. Clinics in Haematology 11(1)
Question 10
Finch C A 1948 Methemoglobin and sulfemoglobin. New England Journal of Medicine 239: 470
Question 11
Goldman J M 1981 Normal leucocytes. In: Hoffbrand A V, Lewis S M (eds) Postgraduate haematology, 2nd edn. William Heinemann, London
Question 12
Videbaek A 1975 Polycythaemia and myelofibrosis. Clinics in Haematology 4(2)
Question 13
Mollison P L, Engelfriet C P, Contreras M 1987 Blood transfusion in clinical medicine, 8th edn. Blackwell, Oxford, ch 7
Question 14
Davidson R J L 1964 Exertional haemoglobinuria: a report on three cases with studies on the haemolytic mechanism. Journal of Clinical Pathology 17: 536
Question 15
Kahler H G, Meynell M J, Cooke W T 1966 Spherocytic anaemia complicated by megaloblastic anaemia of pregnancy. British Medical Journal 1: 779
Question 16
As for MCQ 70, p 71
Question 17
Adams J F, Kennedy E H 1965 Hydroxocobalamin: excretion and retention after parenteral doses in anaemic and non-anaemic subjects, with reference to the treatment of vitamin B_{12} deficiency states. Journal of Laboratory and Clinical Medicine 65: 450
Question 18
Holroet G, Michuelsen P, Vandepitte J 1982 Airport malaria in Belgium. Lancet ii: 881
Question 19
Van der Weyden M, Firkin B G 1972 The management of aplastic anaemia in adults. British Journal of Haematology 22: 1

Question 20
Sharp A A 1977 Diagnosis and management of disseminated intravascular coagulation. British Medical Bulletin 33(3): 265
Question 21
Geary C G, Clough V, MacIver J E 1980 Tropical splenomegaly. British Journal of Hospital Medicine 24: 417
Question 22
Donaldson G W K, Davies S H, Darg A, Richmond J 1969 Coagulation factors in chronic liver disease. Journal of Clinical Pathology 22: 199
Question 23
Giles C, Shuttleworth E M 1958 Megaloblastic anaemia of pregnancy. Lancet ii: 1341
Question 24
Mollison P L, Engelfriet C P, Contreras M 1987 Blood transfusion in clinical medicine, 8th edn. Blackwell, Oxford, ch 8
Question 25
Eichner E R, Hillman R S 1971 The evolution of anaemia in alcoholic patients. American Journal of Medicine 50: 218
Question 26
As for MCQ 70, p 71

3 MRCPath Data Interpretation

Read carefully the clinical and laboratory information provided and answer the questions that follow.

Data Interpretation 1

In a case of disputed paternity the following red cell grouping data was obtained:

	ABO	Rhesus	M	N	S	s	K	k	Fy^a	Fy^b	Jk^a	Jk^b
Mother	B	R_1r	+	+	−	+	−	+	−	+	−	+
Baby	O	R_1r	+	+	−	+	+	+	−	+	+	+
Mr X	A	R_1R_1	+	+	+	−	−	+	−	−	+	+
Mr Y	O	R_2r	−	+	+	+	+	+	+	+	+	+
Mr Z	AB	R_2r''	+	+	−	+	+	+	−	+	−	+

1. What are the characteristics of useful genetic markers for disputed paternity investigation?
2. Which of the three men is most likely to be the baby's father?

Data Interpretation 2

A mother brought her 4-year-old son to the Accident and Emergency department. He had been non-specifically unwell for a week with some vomiting and slightly blood-stained diarrhoea. On the morning of admission he had a convulsion. Other past medical history and family history were non-contributory.

On examination he was pale, dehydrated and ill but fully conscious. A spleen tip was palpable. Pulse 106 beats per minute, BP 120/90, temperature 38.5°C.

Blood count: WBC 14.2 × 10^9/l, Hb 6.2 g/dl, MCV 86, platelets 70 × 10^9/l. Differential: neutrophils 92%, lymphocytes 6%, monocytes 2%. Reticulocytes 16%. Blood film showed burr cells and red cell fragments. Prothrombin time 14 seconds (control 12 seconds) Cerebrospinal fluid was normal apart from a slightly raised protein.

1. What type of anaemia is this?
2. What is the most likely diagnosis?
3. Outline the management of this condition.

Data Interpretation 3

Mr SM is a 68-year-old man who presented with profound haematuria and widespread bruising five days after retropubic prostatectomy. Histology had revealed carcinoma of the prostate but there was no clinical or laboratory evidence of metastatic disease. A coagulation screen showed:

Haemoglobin	10.3 g/dl
Platelets	157 × 10^9/l
Prothrombin time	15 s (control 12 s)
APTT	42 s (control 34 s)
APTT 50/50 mix with normal plasma	35 s
Thrombin time	25 s (control 12 s)
Euglobulin lysis time	43 min (NR 100–280 min)
D-D dimers	6000 ng/ml (NR $<$ 200 ng/ml)

1. Comment on these results.
2. Suggest appropriate therapy to control the bleeding.

Data Interpretation 4

The following results were obtained in three patients' Paul-Bunnell tests. Indicator cells (sheep or horse erythrocytes) have been added to every tube. '+' indicates agglutination, '−' indicates no agglutination.

Dilutions:	Neat	10	40	80	160	320	640
Patient 1							
A	+	+	+	–	–	–	–
B	–	–	–	–	–	–	–
C	+	+	+	–	–	–	–
Patient 2							
A	+	+	+	+	+	+	+
B	+	+	+	+	+	+	+
C	+	+	+	+	–	–	–
Patient 3							
A	+	+	+	+	+	+	+
B	+	+	+	+	–	–	–
C	+	+	+	+	–	–	–

A = patient's serum
B = patient's serum with guinea-pig kidney suspension
C = patient's serum with ox-cell suspension

1. What are the characteristics of the antibody produced in glandular fever?
2. Interpret the results provided.

Data Interpretation 5

A 25-year-old Caucasian woman presented to the Rheumatology Clinic with acute arthritis in both wrists. She had previously been treated with a short course of steroids for thrombocytopenia when 18 and had recently been investigated for over a year for infertility by the Gynaecologists. Haematological investigations were as follows:

Haemoglobin	13.9 g/dl
Platelets	93×10^9/l
Thrombin time	13 s (control 12 s)
Prothrombin time	14 s (control 13 s)
APTT	53 s (control 37 s)
50/50 mixture with normal plasma	58 s
IgM anti-cardiolipin antibody	48.4 M units/ml (Normal range $<$ 15 M units/ml)

Comment on these results and discuss whether there is a risk of excessive bleeding, either spontaneously or following operative procedures, and whether any further haematological tests might be helpful.

Data Interpretation 6

Mrs AH is 25 years old. She is admitted to hospital as an emergency complaining of severe pain and swelling in her shin. She has only been seen at a hospital casualty department on one previous occasion four years before when she developed acute pain in her right shoulder, associated with a chest infection. This resolved spontaneously when she was treated with antibiotics. She describes herself as a fit person and her only problem is occasional attacks of rheumatism which respond to treatment with a mild analgesic.

On examination she is a fit-looking black woman. Her mucous membranes are slightly pale, and apart from a hot, swollen shin there are no physical abnormalities. A full blood count shows a white count of 12.0×10^9/l, haemoglobin of 9.0 g/dl, MCV of 65 fl, a red cell count of 5.6 $\times 10^{12}$/l and a platelet count of 325×10^{12}/l.

1. What is the most likely diagnosis?
2. Name four tests that you would perform.
3. Outline the treatment that you would instigate.

Data Interpretation 7

A 25-year-old woman bled excessively immediately after a normal delivery of a full term baby. The pregnancy had been uneventful except for the finding of moderate leucopenia on a routine blood count performed at 36 weeks. Laboratory findings are as follows:

WBC	3.6×10^9/l, Hb 9.0 g/dl, platelets 70×10^9/l
Differential	neutrophils 20%, lymphocytes 65%, myelocytes 6%, blasts 9%. 6 nucleated red cells/100 WBC.

Prothrombin time	20 s (control 13 s)
APTT	65 s (control 36 s)
Fibrinogen	0.6 g/l
Fibrin degradation products	80–160 μg/ml

1. Discuss the possible diagnoses.
2. Describe the immediate management of the patient.

Data Interpretation 8

A 49-year-old man presents with a two month history of weakness and bone pain. On examination he has hepatosplenomegaly.

Blood count and serum chemistry were as follows: WBC 55×10^9/l, Hb 8.1 g/dl, platelets 65×10^9/l. Differential: neutrophils 10%, lymphocytes 20%, abnormal 'blasts' 70%. Urea 19.0 mmol/l, creatinine 390 μmol/l, calcium 3.24 mmol/l.

A bone marrow was performed, which showed heavy infiltration with blast cells similar to those in the peripheral blood. Routine cytochemistry is unhelpful, but electron microscopy showed the presence of cytoplasmic fibrils. Immunological studies showed that the cells contain cytoplasmic Ig and show positive reaction to the monoclonal antibody OKT 10.

1. What is the diagnosis?
2. What other investigations are indicated?

Data Interpretation 9

A 4-year-old girl of Italian descent presented with acute onset of lethargy and jaundice with dark brown urine. She had spent the previous day on a farm picking fruit and vegetables. On examination she was pale and jaundiced but no other abnormalities were detected. She was apyrexial.

Blood count showed: WBC 12.6×10^9/l, Hb 6.9 g/dl, MCV 104 fl, platelets 450×10^9/l. Differential: neutrophils 80%, lymphocytes 17%, monocytes 3%. Reticulocyte count 28%. Numerous Heinz bodies were seen in the reticulocyte preparation. G6PD spot screening test was normal. Pyruvate kinase assay: 10.9 u/min/ml of red cells (NR 4.5–6.5). G6PD assay: 6.0 iu/g Hb (NR 8–11).

1. Discuss these results.
2. What is the most likely diagnosis?
3. What further investigations would you perform?
4. How would you treat this child?

Data Interpretation 10

A 32-year-old woman was found to have the following blood count at booking in her first pregnancy: WBC 12.8 $\times$ 10^9/l, RBC 4.32 $\times$ 10^{12}/l, PCV 35.1, Hb 12.4 g/dl, MCV 84.2 fl, MCH 28.7 pg, MCHC 35.3 g/dl, RDW 14.2, platelets 92 $\times$ 10^9/l, Pct .123, MPV 13.3, PDW 9.7. Blood film was normal, except for reduced platelets.

At 28 weeks the platelet count was 76 $\times$ 10^9/l, at 36 weeks 52 $\times$ 10^9/l, at 38 weeks 42 $\times$ 10^9/l.

There was no history of hypertension or pre-eclampsia. Ultrasound scan showed normal fetal development. The only drug was Pregaday, one tablet daily.

Bone marrow aspirate demonstrated normal numbers of megakaryocytes and no other abnormality.

1. What is the most likely diagnosis?
2. What treatment would you advise?
3. What is the role of platelet transfusion in this condition?
4. Of what value are platelet parameters MPV and Pct?

Data Interpretation 11

A 40-year-old woman presents in the A&E department with a sudden onset right-sided hemiparesis. She had been admitted to hospital on two previous occasions — with a deep-vein thrombosis of the calf two years previously and an axillary vein thrombosis seven years before. Both had resolved completely after treatment with heparin and warfarin. She stated that she had been feeling listless and tired for the last two years.

On examination she was normotensive and there were no signs of cardiac failure. She was mildly jaundiced.

Blood count showed: WBC 2.6 $\times$ 10^9/l, RBC 3.5 $\times$ 10^{12}/l,

haemoglobin 9.5 g/dl, MCV 70 fl, platelets 250 $\times$ 10^9/l.
Differential neutrophils 25%, lymphocytes 65%, monocytes 10%.
ESR 21 mm/h
ANF negative

1. What is the most likely diagnosis?
2. Name one confirmatory test and three additional tests that you would carry out.
3. Give three approaches to the treatment of this condition.

Data Interpretation 12

A 34-year-old Caucasian woman, para 3 + 1, underwent a caesarian section at 39 weeks because of fetal distress and previous caesarian section. Her pre-operative haemoglobin was 10.4 g/dl, with a normal white cell and platelet count. She received two units of packed cells at elective transfusion on return to the ward, without reaction.

Recovery was uncomplicated until six days after the operation when she suffered a nose bleed and noticed increased bruising at the site of venepunctures.

Blood count showed: WBC 3.7 $\times$ 10^9/l, RBC 4.10 $\times$ 10^{12}/l, Hb 12.2 g/dl, PCV .355, MCV 86.6 fl, MCH 29.8 pg, MCHC 34.4 g/dl, RDW 15.4, platelets 9 $\times$ 10^9/l. Blood film was normal except for thrombocytopenia. Bone marrow aspirate showed increased numbers of megakaryocytes.

1. What is the most likely diagnosis?
2. What is the mechanism of thrombocytopenia in this condition?
3. What treatments are available?

Data Interpretation 13

A 54-year-old woman was noted to be plethoric by her GP, whom she was consulting for a persistent upper respiratory tract infection. There was no significant previous medical history, and she stated that she had always had a high colour.

Physical examination was unremarkable.

Blood count showed: WBC 5.6 $\times$ 10^9/l, RBC 6.44

$\times 10^{12}$/l, Hb 18.6 g/dl, PCV .541, MCV 84 fl, MCH 28.9 pg, MCHC 34.3 g/dl, RDW 10.2, platelets 324 $\times 10^9$/l. Differential: neutrophils 61%, lymphocytes 35%, monocytes 4%. Blood film normal. Neutrophil alkaline phosphatase score 55. Blood gases, urea, MSU, chest X-ray and abdominal ultrasound gave normal results. Haemoglobin oxygen dissociation curve $p^{50} = 12.5$ mmHg.

1. What is the cause of this patient's polycythaemia?
2. What further confirmatory investigations may be performed?
3. What treatment should be given?

Answers/Comments

Data Interpretation Answer 1

In disputed paternity investigations, a very wide range of genetic markers is used. Useful markers must have the following characteristics. Firstly the marker must be maintained from birth to old age (so Lewis, P and I antigens are of no use). Secondly, there must be a single and unequivocal pattern of inheritance. Thirdly, the different phenotypes must be easily distinguishable. Finally, each of the common alleles must have a reasonable frequency. Rare exceptions such as linked phenotypes, recombinations (especially in the HLA system), and variability in antigen expression must be taken into account.

There are two classes of paternity exclusion. A man is excluded if both he and the mother lack an antigen which the baby has (first order exclusion). A man is also excluded if antigens that he must pass on are not present in the child (second order exclusion). Full paternity testing (red cell antigens, HLA typing, red cell iso-enzymes and serum protein types) will give a statistical likelihood of the man not being the father of the child. In this case Mr Y is the most likely father of the child. (See table on p. 103.)

Mr X: First order exclusion — Kell (K)
Second order exclusion — S
Very unlikely to be the father.

Mr Y: First order exclusion — none
Second order exclusion — none
He cannot be excluded on the basis of this limited antigen testing alone. Further testing must be done.

Mr Z: First order exclusion — Jk^a
Second order exclusion — AB (unless he is cis-AB)
— Rh (he must pass on E, which the child does not have)
Again, he is statistically very unlikely to be the father.

In the near future analysis of the patterns produced by cleavage of DNA by restriction endonucleases and electrophoresis followed by hybridisation with gene probes will provide a useful routine method of investigation in cases of disputed paternity.

Data Interpretation Answer 2

The considerable reticulocytosis, red cell morphology and thrombocytopenia are typical of a microangiopathic haemolytic anaemia. The history, haematological findings and clinical features, particularly hypertension, are typical of haemolytic-uraemic syndrome (HUS). The normal prothrombin time makes the diagnosis of disseminated intravascular coagulation most unlikely.

In the management of this condition renal function must be closely monitored as severe oliguric renal failure is common. Therefore urea, creatinine, electrolytes, fluid balance and a daily weight must be checked. Appropriate treatment for renal failure and hypertension must be given. A full clotting screen should be carried out as a baseline, but it is often normal in HUS. A full screen for infection should be performed; HUS may be associated with a variety of infections including respiratory viruses and toxin-producing coliforms, and appropriate treatment must be given where possible. A current hypothesis is that in individuals with

HUS there is an abnormality in prostacyclin metabolism resulting in aggregation of platelets on the vascular endothelium and laying down of fibrin strands. Infusions of fresh frozen plasma are often helpful. These may be combined with plasma exchange if volume overload is a problem or simple infusions ineffective. Other more controversial treatments include vitamin E therapy, heparin and steroids. Once a reasonable platelet count has been achieved anti-platelet agents such as aspirin and Persantin may be administered to prevent aggregation of platelets on the vascular epithelium.

The outlook in HUS has improved, mainly due to the improving management of acute renal failure, but the mortality is still approximately 5%.

Data Interpretation Answer 3

This patient has a prolonged thrombin time and a markedly shortened euglobulin lysis time. The euglobulin lysis time is an overall screening test for the fibrinolytic system, and a shortened time indicates excessive activation of the fibrinolytic system. This usually occurs secondary to acute DIC but primary hyperfibrinolysis may develop in certain forms of gynaecological, post-dental extraction and post-prostatectomy bleeding. Localised and subsequently systemic release of plasminogen activators (often present in prostatic carcinoma tissue), causes fibrin digestion leading to the formation of fibrin degradation products and hypofibrinogenaemia. Latex agglutination tests for FDPs are relatively non-specific and raised D-D dimer levels, (formed by the lysis of cross-linked fibrin strands), is a test which is becoming widely available, are suggestive of specific fibrin breakdown. Excessive primary fibrinolysis can be corrected by therapy with EACA or tranexamic acid which are specific inhibitors of plasminogen activators.

Data Interpretation Answer 4

The antibody produced in glandular fever is a heterophile antibody (it reacts with the cells of other animal species) of IgM type. It will be adsorbed by ox red cells but will not be adsorbed by guinea-pig kidney cells. It will agglutinate sheep and horse red cells.

Patient 1 shows the pattern of a normal individual. This shows the activity of the Forsmann antibody — a normal, naturally occurring heterophile antibody reacting with a wide variety of animal tissues.

Patient 2 has glandular fever with a high-titre antibody. The patient's serum agglutinates the indicator cells to a high titre; this agglutination still occurs when the serum is mixed with guinea-pig kidney cells as the antibody is not adsorbed by these cells. However, the antibody is partially adsorbed (to at least a two-tube difference compared to untreated serum) by ox red blood cells.

Patient 3 shows the typical pattern seen in serum sickness following a therapeutic injection of horse derived protein. The individual has developed heterophile antibodies to a high titre that agglutinate the indicator erythrocytes; this antibody is partially adsorbed by both the guinea-pig and the ox tissue.

Data Interpretation Answer 5

This patient has a markedly prolonged APTT and a mild degree of thrombocytopenia. The absence of any significant correction of the prolonged APTT after a 1:1 (50:50) with normal plasma is suggestive of the presence of an inhibitor. From the clinical history, presence of thrombocytopenia and a raised cardiolipin antibody level, this inhibitor is most likely to be a lupus-type anticoagulant. Lupus anticoagulants are directed against phospholipids so non-specifically prolong the APTT and occasionally the prothrombin time of normal plasma. They do not specifically inactivate any of the clotting factors but inhibit prothrombin activation in phospholipid-dependent tests. Thrombocytopenia co-exists with the anticoagulant in a significant number of patients due to cross reactivity of the phospholipid causing premature peripheral platelet destruction and an immune type thrombocytopenia. The lupus anticoagulant and a prolonged APTT do not predispose to clinical bleeding events, and only if associated with a platelet count $< 50 \times 10^9/l$ do specific precautions need to be taken. Similarly the majority of patients have raised levels of anti-cardiolipin antibodies due to the anti-phospholipid nature of the antibody. The lupus anticoagulant is associated with an increased incidence of venous and arterial thrombotic episodes, infertility and recurrent abortions. In selected cases steroid therapy may lead to a disappearance of the inhibitor effect.

Data Interpretation Answer 6

The fact that this woman is black raises the possibility of a sickle cell crisis. Her low MCV and high red cell count suggest thalassaemia so the possibility of sickle thalassaemia should be considered. She needs a sickle solubility screen, haemoglobin electrophoresis, serum ferritin, and X-rays of her affected joints and of her shoulders, hands and hips.

Treatment for a sickle cell crisis involves analgesia, rehydration and antibiotic therapy as indicated. This woman turned out, on sickle cell screening and haemoglobin electrophoresis, to suffer from sickle β-thalassaemia, although she had been relatively little bothered by her disease before. She was admitted for bed-rest and rehydration and, although she remained apyrexial, commenced on antibiotics to cover the possibility of osteomyelitis.

Data Interpretation Answer 7

This young woman has a leucoerythroblastic blood film, thrombocytopenia, and evidence of disseminated intravascular coagulation (DIC). The presence of leucopenia with a relatively high proportion of blasts makes a primary haematological malignancy more likely than reactive changes secondary to the blood loss. There is no history of abruption, sepsis or pre-eclampsia to account for the DIC, and the most likely explanation is that she has DIC secondary to acute leukaemia, with M3 (acute promyelocytic leukaemia) the most likely type.

Immediate management should include treatment of the bleeding problems with fresh frozen plasma, cryoprecipitate and platelets as necessary. Heparin therapy in DIC is controversial but should be given in M3 AML when starting cytotoxic therapy. A suitable dose is 100 units an hour by continuous intravenous infusion. The diagnosis of M3 AML should be confirmed by bone marrow examination. The presence of a (15,17) chromosome translocation would be useful supportive evidence.

Data Interpretation Answer 8

This relatively young man has anaemia, hepatosplenomegaly, a leukaemic blood picture, renal impairment and hypercalcaemia.

The blast cells have features of late B cells or plasma cells and contain cytoplasmic fibrils characteristic of plasma cells. The likely diagnosis is therefore plasma cell leukaemia. His bone pain is probably related to skeletal deposits. Additional investigations may include further immunological studies on the abnormal cells, using specific monoclonal antibodies, assessment of any paraprotein and urinary light chain excretion, and measurement of immunoglobulin levels. Radiological assessment of bone involvement, plasma viscosity and further assessment of renal function may also be performed.

Data Interpretation Answer 9

This girl has had an acute haemolytic crisis and the blood film shows evidence of oxidative damage to haemoglobin (Heinz bodies). An unstable haemoglobin is possible but the most likely diagnosis is glucose-6-phosphate dehydrogenase (G6PD) deficiency with favism. Favism is the extreme hypersensitivity to divisin (found in fava beans and pollen) that occurs particularly in the Mediterranean form of G6PD deficiency. The G6PD genes are carried on the X chromosome and clinical deficiency is therefore seen most commonly in males. However, due to Lyonisation of the X chromosome a heterozygous female has one population of normal red blood cells and one population of deficient red cells. The ratio of normal to deficient red cells is on average 50:50 but this can be very variable, with some individuals having 70% abnormal cells. These females are particularly likely to exhibit clinical manifestations of their deficiency state. In this patient the G6PD spot screening test was normal, reflecting a level only just below the normal range. This level is, however, quite significantly reduced when it is appreciated that there is a 28% reticulocytosis, as young red cells contain higher levels of G6PD. The high level of pyruvate kinase similarly reflects the reticulocytosis.

The diagnosis of G6PD heterozygosity can be confirmed by cytochemical staining of the red cell for G6PD activity. This revealed that 30% of the red cells were G6PD deficient but in the steady state this figure rose to 65%. Family studies may also be of value. In a fit 4-year-old child with a haemoglobin of 6.9 g/dl careful observation only is required. In male children the haemoglobin may fall quite precipitously. The Mediterranean variant of G6PD deficiency is not self-limiting and transfusion may be required. Advice should be given about avoidance of fava beans and oxidant drugs and prompt treatment of infections.

Data Interpretation Answer 10

Idiopathic (auto-immune) thrombocytopenic purpura (ITP) is the most likely diagnosis.

The most appropriate treatment is either high purity intravenous IgG gammaglobulin 0.4 g/kg daily for three days and/or prednisolone 1 mg/kg p.o. daily. Intravenous gammaglobulin produces a rise in platelet count within three days in the majority of cases. The aim is to produce a haemostatic platelet count for delivery. Immediately on delivery the baby's platelet count should be checked as some maternal platelet antibodies cross the placenta, causing neonatal thrombocytopenia. Some authorities have urged delivery by caesarian section as being less traumatic to the baby.

In ITP, platelet transfusions should be reserved for the management of life-threatening bleeding and to cover for operations when the platelet count is less than 50×10^9/l. The transfused platelets are likely to be destroyed by the same immune process causing the thrombocytopenia, and may stimulate the production of platelet allo-antibodies, so that when platelet transfusion is desperately indicated they are ineffective.

In a case of thrombocytopenia, an elevated MPV (mean platelet volume) suggests the reason is peripheral destruction of platelets rather than marrow underproduction. Plateletcrit (Pct) may be a more accurate guide to bleeding tendency than the platelet count, as the ability to plug capillary holes may relate more to platelet mass per volume of blood than to absolute platelet numbers.

Data Interpretation Answer 11

The features of repeated venous thrombosis, iron deficiency anaemia and neutropenia are highly suggestive of paroxysmal nocturnal haemoglobinuria (PNH). Disseminated malignancy should also be considered, but the long history, marked neutropenia, and normal ESR make this unlikely. The negative ANF and normal ESR make a diagnosis of systemic lupus erythematosus unlikely.

The confirmatory test for PNH is the Ham's acid serum haemolysis test. This demonstrates that a population of the patient's red cells are abnormally sensitive to lysis by complement in an acid environment. Other useful tests would include serum iron/TIBC or ferritin to confirm iron deficiency, haemoglobin A_2 estimation to exclude β-thalassaemia trait, serum haptoglobin level to confirm haemolysis and a direct antiglobulin test to exclude auto-immune haemolytic anaemia.

Treatment with corticosteroids may abolish the haemolysis in PNH. Androgen therapy may also be beneficial. Blood transfusion may be necessary but washed red cells should be used as the complement present in normal stored blood may induce lysis if transfused to patients with PNH. Bone marrow transplantation from a matched sibling donor is a therapeutic option, but many patients with PNH are too old at presentation, or do not have a suitable donor.

Data Interpretation Answer 12

The most likely diagnosis is post-transfusion purpura (PTP). This condition is rare but the history in this case is typical. PTP occurs in individuals who are negative for a very common platelet-specific antigen Pl^{A1}. These individuals will have been exposed to the Pl^{A1} antigen before — either from previous blood transfusion or a fetal–maternal leak from a Pl^{A1} positive fetus. This stimulates the formation of anti-Pl^{A1} antibodies. The later transfusion of Pl^{A1} positive blood to an individual with anti-Pl^{A1} antibodies results in thrombocytopenia, often severe, about a week later. It is thought that the patient's own Pl^{A1} negative platelets are destroyed via an 'innocent-bystander' reaction when the transfused platelets form immune complexes with the anti-Pl^{A1}.

Exchange transfusion has proved to be an effective treatment. Random platelet transfusion is ineffectual and may be associated with severe reactions, but some blood transfusion centres may be able to supply platelet concentrate from Pl^{A1}-negative donors. High-purity intravenous IgG gammaglobulin has been used with some success in PTP.

Data Interpretation Answer 13

The most likely cause of this patient's polycythaemia is a high affinity haemoglobin. Because of a structural abnormality of the haemoglobin molecule, oxygen is not easily released to the tissues and tissue hypoxia leads to increased erythropoietin production which stimulates bone marrow erythropoiesis. This is represented by a left shift of the oxygen dissociation curve (Fig. 3.1). The p^{50} is the oxygen tension at which the haemoglobin is 50% saturated.

Haemoglobin electrophoresis will usually show an abnormal band, although different pHs may need to be used. Family studies may be performed to demonstrate an inheritance that is usually autosomal dominant.

Generally these patients require no treatment and live a normal life span. However, should they become pregnant the incidence of miscarriage is high because the abnormal

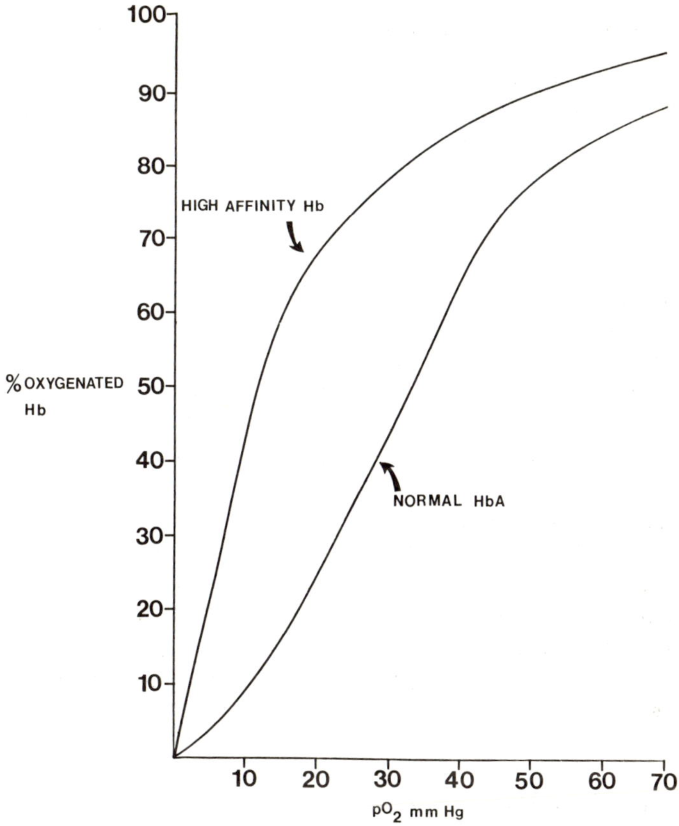

Fig. 3.1 Oxygen dissociation curve of normal and high affinity haemoglobin. The latter is shifted to the left — for a given pO_2 the haemoglobin molecule holds more oxygen — resulting in relative tissue hypoxia and compensatory polycythaemia.

haemoglobin does not easily release oxygen to the tissues. It is not known whether any specific therapy is helpful in this situation, and the use of venesection is controversial.

FURTHER READING

Question 1
Race R R, Sanger R 1975 Blood groups in man, 6th edn. Blackwell Scientific Publications, Oxford

Question 2
Lieberman E 1972 Hemolytic uremic syndrome. Journal of Pediatrics 80: 1

Question 3
Kernoff P B A, McNichol G P 1970 Normal and abnormal fibrinolysis. British Medical Bulletin 34: 129
Question 4
Evans A S, Niederman J C, Cenabre L C, West B, Richards V A 1975 Specificity, sensitivity, and persistence of heterophile and EB-virus specific IgM antibodies in clinical and subclinical infectious mononucleosis. Journal of Infectious Diseases 132: 546
Question 5
Lechner K 1974 Acquired inhibitors in nonhemophilic patients. Haemostasis 3: 65
Question 6
Charache S 1981 Treatment of sickle cell anaemia. Annual Review of Medicine 32: 195
Question 7
Groopman J, Ellman J 1979 Acute promyelocytic leukaemia. American Journal of Hematology 7: 395
Rowley J D, Golomb H M, Dougherty C 1977 15/17 translocation, a consistent chromosomal change in acute promyelocytic leukaemia. Lancet i: 549
Question 8
Parreira et al 1985 Primary plasma cell leukaemia: immunological and ultrastructural studies in 6 cases. Scandinavian Journal of Haematology 35(5): 570
Question 9
Luzatto L 1975 Inherited haemolytic states: glucose 6 phosphate dehydrogenase deficiency. Clinics in Haematology 4: 83
Question 10
Carloss H W, McMillan R, Crosby W H 1980 Management of pregnancy in women with immune thrombocytopenic purpura. Journal of the American Medical Association 224: 2756
Question 11
Sirchia G, Lewis S M 1975 Paroxysmal nocturnal haemoglobinuria. Clinics in Haematology 4(1): 199
Question 12
Abramson M, Eisenberg P D, Aster R H 1974 Post-transfusion purpura: immunologic aspects and therapy. New England Journal of Medicine 291: 1163
Question 13
Weatherall D J 1969 Polycythaemia resulting from abnormal hemoglobins. New England Journal of Medicine 280: 604

4 MRCPath Long Cases

Read carefully the history and investigations on each case and answer the questions that follow.

Long Case 1

Miss AS, a 23-year-old night club hostess was referred pre-operatively because of a history of easy bruising. In 1978 she had undergone surgery for a haemorrhagic cyst of the ovary and since then had had several gynaecological consultations for irregular and heavy periods. She was not receiving any medication and the gynaecologists were planning to do a D&C.

On examination she had several bruises on the thighs, upper arms and neck which were suggestive of recent mild trauma.

Investigations showed:

Haemoglobin	13.4 g/dl
Platelets	415×10^9/l
Bleeding time (template)	13 min
Prothrombin time	12 s (control 12 s)
APTT	38 s (control 36 s)
Thrombin time	12 s (control 12 s)

Platelet aggregation studies were performed and a copy of the traces obtained is shown in Figures 4.1–4.3

Platelet nucleotides (nM/10^9 platelets)
Total content:

ATP	13.8	(NR 16–36)
ADP	2.3	(NR 6.2–12.2)
Ratio	6.0	

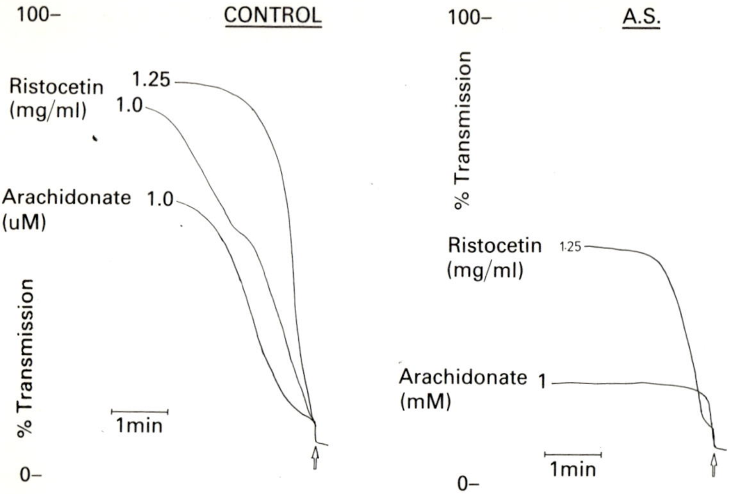

Fig. 4.1 Platelet aggregation curves from a normal control and patient A S in response to ristocetin and arachidonic acid.

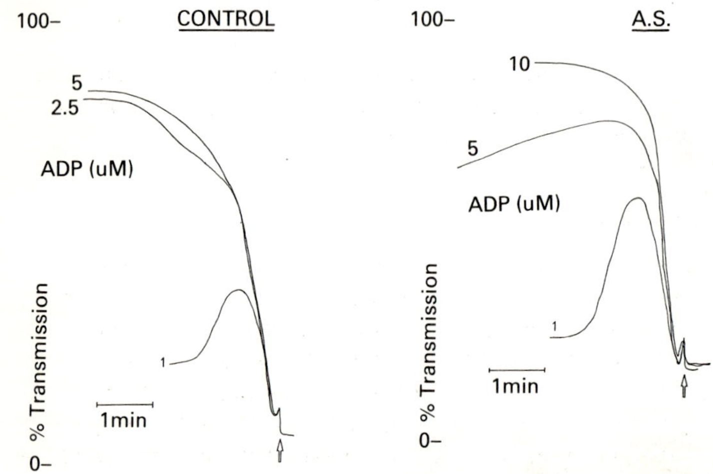

Fig. 4.2 Platelet aggregation curves from a normal control and patient A S in response to various concentrations of ADP.

Release to 20 μg/ml collagen:

ATP	0.9	(NR 1.3–4.9)
ADP	1.2	(NR 2.6–6.6)

Ratio: 0.75

13% of nucleotides released

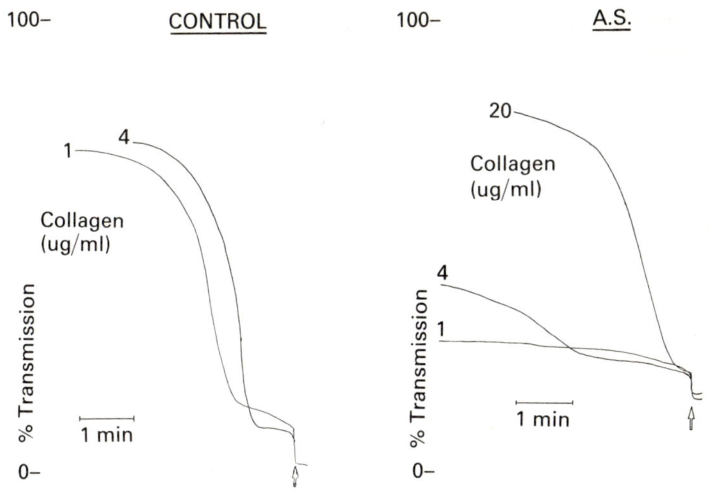

Fig. 4.3 Platelet aggregation curves from a normal control and patient A S in response to various concentrations of collagen.

Report on these findings as if you were the Consultant Haematologist and comment on how you would manage this patient during the operative period.

Long Case 2

A 26-year-old man was admitted for renal transplantation. He had had a ileal conduit operation performed when aged 18 months because of anatomical abnormalities of his renal tract. A succession of further operations had failed to prevent the onset of end-stage renal failure, and he had commenced haemodialysis a year before. He had required numerous transfusions for his operations, but pre-operative screen for atypical red cell antibodies was negative.

Tissue typing of his immediate family had shown his father to be the closest match, and he donated a kidney. During the transplant operation the patient required a two unit blood transfusion. Post-operatively he was started on cyclosporin and anti-lymphocyte globulin. Two weeks after the operation a further cross-match was requested for a two unit top-up transfusion.

Routine cross-match showed both units to be incompatible by the indirect antiglobulin technique.

Repeat blood group: A_2 Rh positive

Auto direct antiglobulin test: positive with IgG. Cell panel using 12 typed group O cells was negative.

What further information do you require, what further investigations should be performed, and how would you manage this patient's transfusion?

Long Case 3

A 10-year-old girl presented with a three-week history of general malaise and sore throat. Examination revealed generalised shotty (< 1 cm) lymphadenopathy and a just palpable spleen. A chest X-ray was normal. A blood count revealed:

Haemoglobin	10.6 g/dl
WBC	$11.1 \times 10^9/l$
Platelets	$160 \times 10^9/l$
Differential:	neutrophils 12%, lymphocytes 35%, monocytes 2%, blast cells 51%.

The bone marrow was hypercellular and contained 80% blasts. Peripheral blood mononuclear cells were isolated and the membrane phenotype determined by indirect immunoflourescence:

Anti-CD2 (T11)	38%
Anti-CD3 (T3)	34%
Anti-CD4 (T4)	21%
Anti-CD8 (T8)	13%
Anti-CD6 (T6)	0%
Anti-CALLA	49%
Anti-HLA-DR	58%
Anti-surface immunoglobulin	2%
Anti-myeloid antibody	2%

Discuss the phenotype results and their prognostic significance.

Long Case 4

MS is an 8-year-old girl from South America. She has apparently suffered from anaemia all her life and requires, according to the mother's history, a blood transfusion of approximately two units every four weeks. She is said to be suffering from thalassaemia major. Apart from becoming tired prior to transfusion she has always been reasonably fit.

On examination she is a pale thin child who is on the 50 percentile for height and 60 percentile for weight. There is no hepatosplenomegaly, and she has a normal facies.

Blood count showed: WBC 5.5 $\times 10^9$/l, RBC 2.65 $\times 10^{12}$/l, Hb 7.0 g/dl, MCV 98 fl, platelets 400 $\times 10^9$/l.

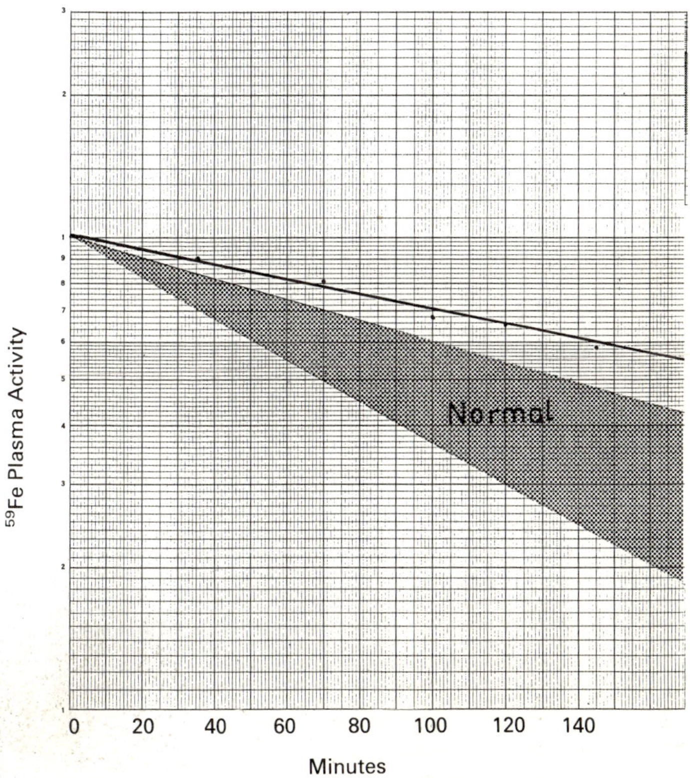

Fig. 4.4 ^{59}Fe plasma iron clearance. The normal range is shaded.

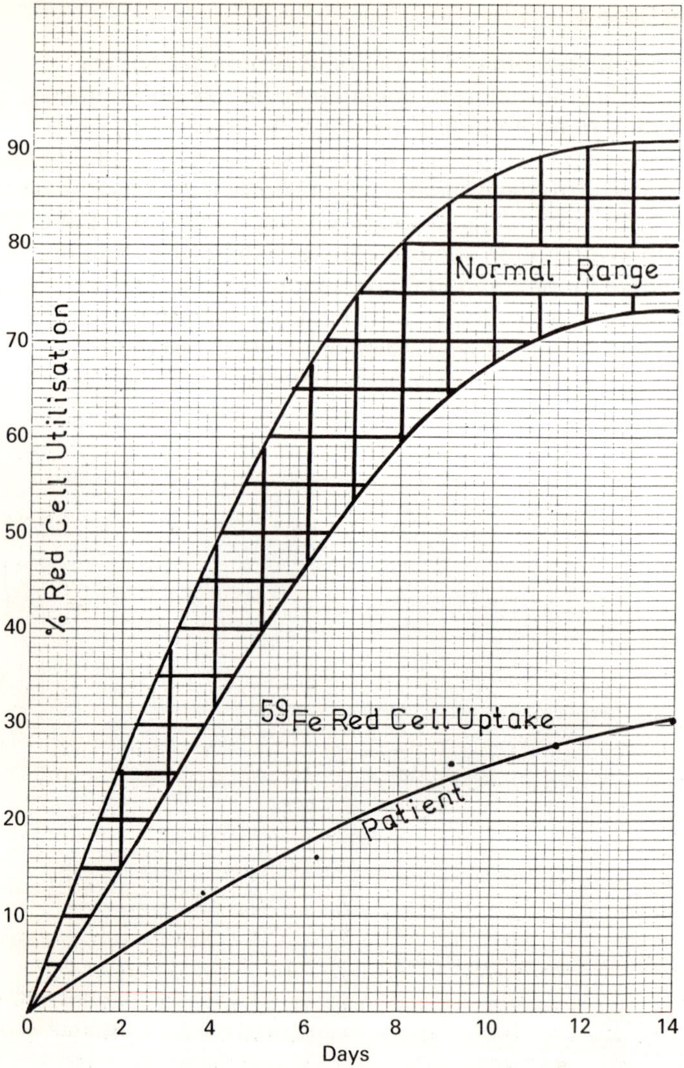

Fig. 4.5 ^{59}Fe red cell iron uptake. The normal range is shaded.

1. What are the possible diagnoses? Explain your choices.
2. What investigations would you request?
3. Interpret this patient's iron utilisation curve (Fig. 4.4), and red cell iron uptake (Fig. 4.5). Use these to make your final diagnosis.

Long Case 5

A 21-year-old woman of Turkish descent attended the antenatal clinic for the first time at 24 weeks of pregnancy. She felt well and examination revealed that she had an appropriately sized fetus. She was noted to be rather pale.

Blood count showed: WBC $3.6 \times 10^9/l$, Hb 8.4 g/dl, MCV 71 fl, RDW 29.6, platelets $167 \times 10^9/l$. Differential count: neutrophils 62%, lymphocytes 37%, monocytes 1%. Blood film showed marked anisocytosis, and occasional neutrophil hypersegmentation.

Further investigations were performed: serum iron 10 μmol/l, TIBC 65 μmol/l, B_{12} 150 pg/ml (NR 150–700), red cell folate 57 ng/ml (NR 150–700). Haemoglobin electrophoresis: predominantly HbA, HbA_2 1.0%, HbF 1.1%. A fast band is present is small quantities.

Discuss the likely diagnosis and the management of this case.

Long Case 6

A 75-year-old woman presented with lumps in the neck and shortness of breath on exercise.

On examination she had 2 cm nodes palpable in both sides of the neck and both axillae. The spleen was just palpable.

Blood count showed: WBC $71.0 \times 10^9/l$, RBC $2.9 \times 10^{12}/l$, Hb 8.6 g/dl, PCV .291, MCV 100 fl, MCH 29.6, platelets $160 \times 10^9/l$. Differential: neutrophils 5%, lymphocytes 94%, monocytes 1%. Film examination: shows anisocytosis and polychromasia. Reticulocyte count: 7%.

She was treated with chlorambucil and prednisolone for six months and the lymph nodes became much smaller, the spleen impalpable, and the white count fell to $14 \times 10^9/l$. Therapy was then stopped.

Two years later she was admitted via the A&E department with acute abdominal pain. On examination she had 1 cm lymphadenopathy in the neck and axillae. In the abdomen there was guarding and rebound tenderness in the umbilical area. The liver was 3 cm enlarged and the spleen 6 cm enlarged.

The blood count showed: WBC 30 × 10^9/l, Hb 12.0 g/dl, platelets 210 × 10^9/l. Differential: neutrophils 26%, lymphocytes 72%, monocytes 2%.

A laparotomy was performed and three perforations of the small bowel were found and resected. Around these segments of bowel were matted lymph nodes. Large mesenteric and para-aortic glands were also found.

1. What was the full diagnosis at presentation?
2. What is the likely diagnosis now? Discuss your further management of the case.

Long Case 7

A 59-year-old Caucasian woman presented with painful, red eyes and a 'flushed face'.

On examination marked venous congestion of the conjunctiva and retina was found. The spleen was just palpable. Her weight was 50 kg.

Blood count showed: WBC 16.0 × 10^9/l, RBC 6.93 × 10^{12}/l, Hb 19.0 g/dl, PCV .651, MCV 93 fl, MCH 27.4 pg. Red cell mass by Cr^{51}-labelled red cell method: 1.9 litres.

1. Comment on the investigations performed so far.

Treatment was commenced with venesection and ^{32}P, and the patient remained well for six years. Her spleen then enlarged to 16 cm and caused severe discomfort, and she also became transfusion-dependent.

Blood count at this time showed: WBC 15 × 10^9/l, Hb 7.1 g/dl, platelets 36 × 10^9/l.

Radioisotopic studies were performed, shown in Figures 4.6 and 4.7

2. Comment on the investigations performed.

Six months later she again required transfusion. Blood count at this time showed: WBC 97 × 10^9/l, Hb 8.2 g/dl, platelets 46 × 10^9/l. Differential: granulocytic cells 73%, lymphocytes 4%, monocytes 4%, blast cells 19%

3. Comment on the diagnosis at this stage and say how you would manage this woman.

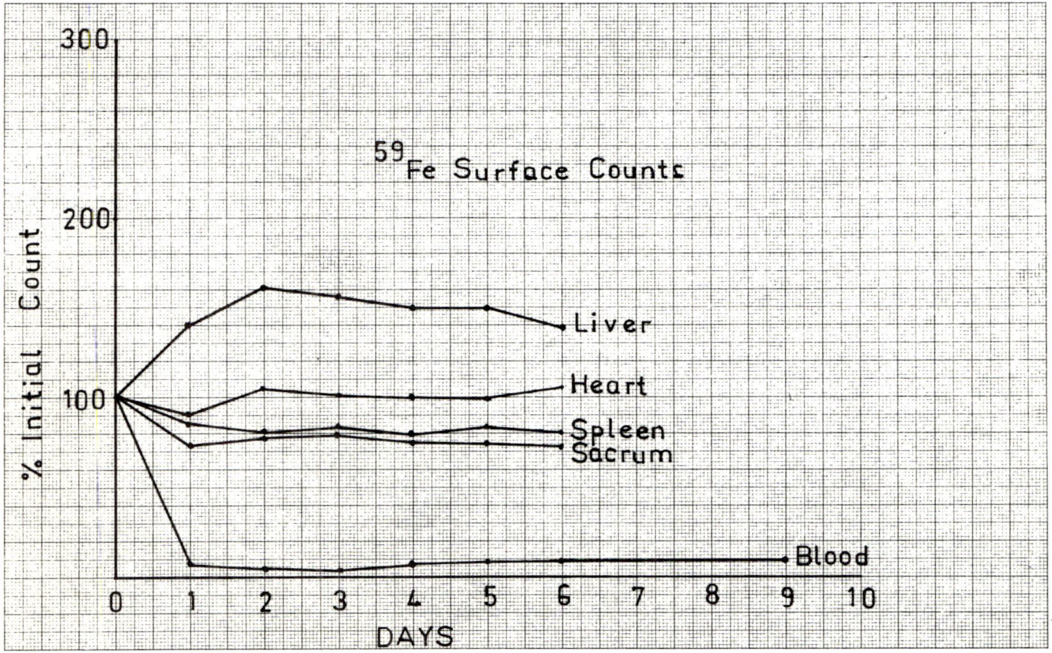

Fig. 4.6 ^{59}Fe surface counting over liver, heart, spleen, and sacrum. Blood activity is also shown. These are expressed as a percentage on initial readings.

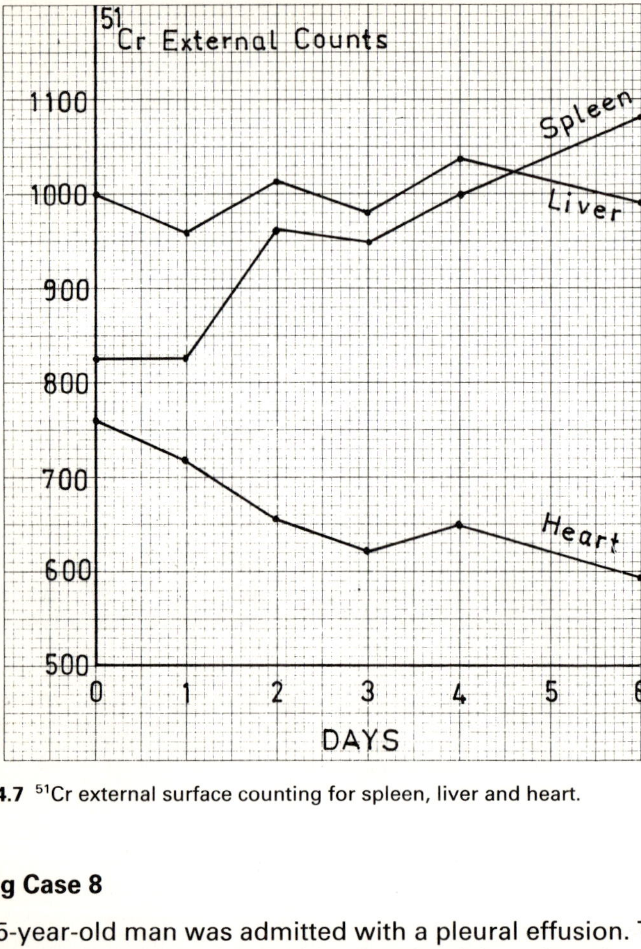

Fig. 4.7 ^{51}Cr external surface counting for spleen, liver and heart.

Long Case 8

A 75-year-old man was admitted with a pleural effusion. This was tapped and found to be blood-stained, but pleural biopsy showed no evidence of malignancy. A provisional diagnosis of pulmonary infarction is made.

Ten years before he had had a partial gastrectomy at which time his spleen was removed for technical reasons. He had no recent gastrointestinal symptoms, but he had had a myocardial infarction six months ago at which time he was noted to have a moderate leucocytosis and thrombocytosis. The SHO was worried about his blood count and wondered if he may have some kind of leukaemia. He asked your advice.

The most recent blood count was: WBC 37.7 × 10^9/l, Hb

12.6 g/dl, platelets 1142 × 10^9/l. Differential: neutrophils 74%, lymphocytes 10%, monocytes 10%, eosinophils 3%, myelocytes 1%. Blood film: target cells, Howell-Jolly bodies, giant platelets and megakaryocyte fragments.

Advise regarding further investigations and possible diagnoses.

Long Case 9

A 54-year-old man developed excessive bleeding from the chest drainage tubes six hours after cardiac bypass surgery for a triple vein graft. The bleeding was at a steady rate of approximately 100 ml/hour from each of the two drains, and there was excessive bruising around the central line insertion site and at the sites of two recent femoral blood gas aspiration sites.

A coagulation screen was performed. The results of this, the pre-operative screen, and the screen performed immediately after heparin reversal (fifteen minutes after completion of the operation) are shown in the table below.

	Pre-operative	*15 minutes postoperatively*	*6 hours later*	*Normal range*
Hb (g/dl)	14.7	9.3	7.4	
Haematocrit	0.48	0.31	0.23	
Platelets (× 10^9/l)	323	107	113	
Prothrombin time (s)	14	15	15	12–16
Thrombin time (s)	12	19	120	11–14
APTT (s)	38	43	120	30–40
Fibrinogen (g/dl)	2.7	1.8	1.9	1.5–4.0
Thrombin time with 1 mg % protamine (s)	—	—	19	11–15

Comment on the findings and advise on the future management of this patient.

Long Case 10

A female baby of Indian extraction was born at term by normal delivery. One hour after birth 1 mg of prophylactic vitamin K was given by intramuscular injection. The following day an enlarging thigh haematoma appeared at the site of the injection, heel-prick sites started to bleed and petechiae developed over the left shoulder and lower abdomen.

The results of a coagulation screen were as follows:

Haemoglobin	13.1 g/dl
Platelets	152×10^9/l
Template bleeding time	9 min
APTT	120 s (NR 30–40 s)
Prothrombin time	180 s (NR 12–16)
Thrombin time	17 s (NR 10–12)
Stypven time	120 s (NR 15–18)

Prothrombin time corrections:

80% patient's plasma + 20% normal plasma	20 s
80% patient's plasma + 20% Al $(OH)_2$ adsorbed plasma	86 s
80% patient's plasma + 20% normal serum	18 s

Report on these findings. How would you manage the child's bleeding tendency?

Long Case 11

A 49-year-old Caucasian woman was referred by the dermatologists with a history of Raynaud's phenomenon and livedo reticularis since the age of 14. She had two pregnancies, both of which resulted in stillbirths, and she had developed deep-vein thromboses after both pregnancies. Following a hysterectomy when aged 45 she had a severe postoperative haemorrhage which required a four unit blood transfusion. She again developed an extensive deep-vein thrombosis in her left leg and a post-phlebitic leg ulcer.

The results of her coagulation studies were as follows:

Liver function tests	within normal limits
Platelet count	166×10^9/l
Bleeding time (template)	6 min
Prothrombin time	15 s (NR 12–14 s)
APTT	42 s (NR 30–40 s)
APTT 50/50 mix with normal plasma	35 s
Thrombin time	> 180 s (NR 12–14 s)
Thrombin time with 10 mg % protamine sulphate	> 60 s
Reptilase time	30 s (NR 16–18 s)

Fibrinogen (clot weight)	0.58 g/l
Fibrinogen (Clauss)	0.24 g/l
Fibrinogen (RAg)	0.94 g/l
AT III (chromogenic assay)	83% (NR 80–120%)

Comment on these results and outline your management of this case.

Long Case 12

Mr GL, an 81-year-old Caucasian man, was referred from another hospital after continual bleeding from an operative incision. 20 days before he had had an inguinal hernia repaired but because of continuing blood loss from the wound he had been re-explored five times and had had to undergo orchidectomy because of an enlarging scrotal haematoma.

On admission the coagulation screen showed:

Haemoglobin	10.1 g/dl
Platelets	323×10^9/l
Bleeding time (template)	> 20 min
Prothrombin time	16 s (NR 12–16 s)
APTT	59 s (NR 30–40 s)
APTT with 50% normal plasma	49 s
Thrombin time	16 s (control 12–14 s)
Factor VIII:C	0.11 iu/ml (NR 0.5–2.0 iu/ml)
Factor VIII:vWF	< 0.02 iu/ml (NR 0.5–2.0 iu/ml)
Factor VIII:vWFag	< 0.02 iu/ml (NR 0.5–2.0 iu/ml)
Bethesda inhibitor assay to factor VIII:C	negative

An infusion of 50 units of cryoprecipitate was then given and a five minute post-infusion sample tested:

APTT	44 s
Factor VIII:C	0.29 iu/ml
Factor VIII:vWF	< 0.02 iu/ml
Bleeding time (template)	18 min

Report on these findings and discuss the management of this patient.

Long Case 13

An orthopaedic surgeon referred a patient to the haematology clinic with a request for autotransfusion. The patient was a 49-year-old woman with a 20-year history of sero-positive erosive rheumatoid arthritis. Previous treatment for her arthritis had included gold, penicillamine, indomethacin and prednisolone. Her symptoms had been controlled recently by enteric-coated aspirin and piroxicam. Eight years before she had had a bilateral knee replacement with the uneventful transfusion of eight units of blood. Four years ago she had had a left hip replacement with the transfusion of three units of blood. A further cross-match has been requested for four units, but all four are incompatible by the indirect antiglobulin technique. Blood group is O Rh positive. The patient's serum reacted with all cells of a 12 cell commercial antibody identification panel by the indirect antiglobulin technique.

Blood count shows: WBC 7.8×10^9/l, RBC 4.23×10^{12}/l, Hb 8.9 g/dl, Hct .292, MCV 69 fl, MCH 21.0 pg, MCHC 30.5 g/dl, RDW 18.8, platelets 576×10^9/l. ESR 120 mm/h. Serum ferritin 29 μg/ml, serum iron 11 mmol/l, TIBC 35 mmol/l. Red cell folate 240 μg/l (normal 150–650).

1. Is she suitable for autotransfusion?
2. Outline further investigations that you would perform.

The serum was referred to the Regional Blood Transfusion Centre for testing against a panel of cells lacking common public antigens. This allowed identification of anti-v, anti-Yk^a (York), and anti-Kn^a (Knopps-Holgerson) antibodies. The v (ce^s) antigen has an incidence of 0.4% in Caucasians and 40% in blacks. Review of the literature showed that both anti-Kn^a and anti-Yk^a have been reported as a cause of transfusion reactions. However normal in vivo survival of Yk^{a+} cells has also been reported.

3. What are the possible options for obtaining blood for her operation?

Two units of v negative blood were selected and red cells from the pilot tube were labelled with ^{51}Cr and injected into the patient. Blood samples were taken over the following three weeks. A survival curve was plotted (see Fig. 4.8).

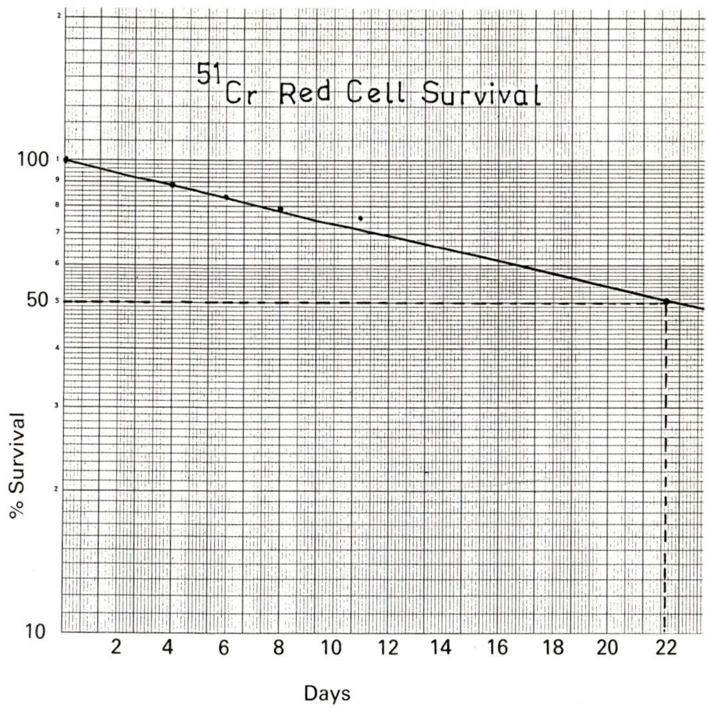

Fig. 4.8 ^{51}Cr red cell survival for Long Case 13.

4. Advise on the in vivo compatibility of these units of blood.

Long Case 14

A 34-year-old man of mixed race had a four month history of tiredness, anorexia and weight loss. He had slightly increased bowel frequency and some generalised abdominal discomfort. He had also noted pains in his hands and feet. His diet was normal.

On examination the positive findings were pallor, prematurely grey hair and a smooth sore tongue.

Blood count showed: WBC $2.7 \times 10^9/l$, RBC 3.06 $\times 10^{12}/l$, Hb 7.6 g/dl, PCV .248, MCV 81 fl, MCH 24.8 pg. Differential: neutrophils 48%, lymphocytes 46%, monocytes

4%, eosinophils 2%. Blood and bone marrow films are shown below in Figures 4.9a and 4.9b.

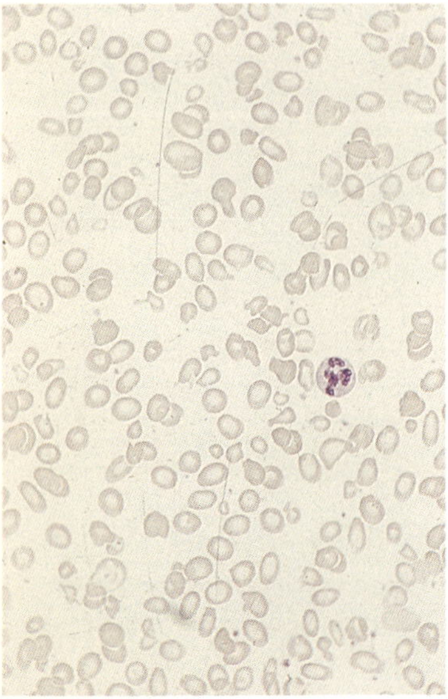

Fig. 4.9a Blood

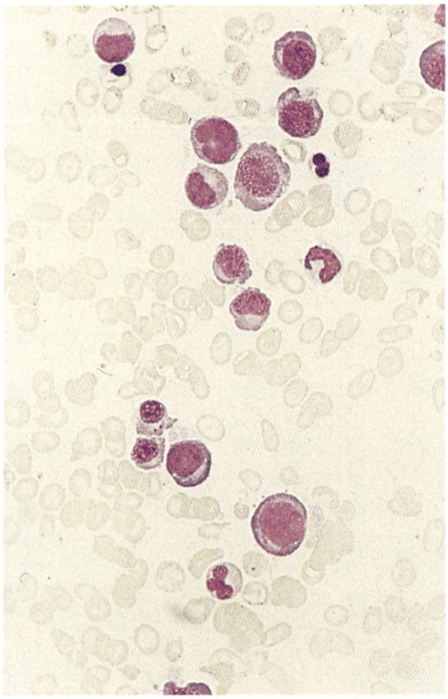

Fig. 4.9b Bone marrow

1. Comment on the haematological findings and outline the further investigations that you require.

Further investigations, with their results, are as follows: Liver function tests: bilirubin 26 μmol/l (NR 1–17), AST 24 iu/l (NR < 40), alkaline phosphatase 146 (NR < 300), total protein 70 g/l, albumin 47 g/l. Serum B_{12} and folate: B_{12} 15 ng/l, serum folate 5.0 μg/l, red cell folate 45 μg/l. Haemoglobin electrophoresis: haemoglobin A major band, HbA_2 5.8%, HbF 1.2%

2. What is the diagnosis?
3. What further investigations are required?

A Schilling test showed 8% excretion in part I, and 9% in part II.

4. What further investigations should be performed?

Answers/Comments

Long Case Answer 1

The patient has a prolonged bleeding time, but a normal platelet count and coagulation screen. These results, in the presence of no obvious clinical features of a vascular defect and normal haematocrit levels, are suggestive of a platelet function defect. Before proceeding with further investigations it is important to ensure that the patient has not ingested any drugs over the last 7–10 days, (particularly aspirin and non-steroidal anti-inflammatory agents), which could interfere with platelet function and prolong the bleeding time.

Platelet studies in platelet-rich plasma revealed markedly impaired responses to low-dose (1 and 4 μg/ml) collagen, a reversible primary wave only with 5 mM ADP and an absent response to arachidonic acid. Platelet nucleotide quantitation showed a reduced total content of ATP and ADP. This technique measures both the metabolic and dense granule pool of nucleotides. Upon maximal stimulation with 20 μg/ml collagen the release of the dense granule contents are specifically assessed and these were also markedly reduced. These findings suggest the diagnosis of a storage pool defect (SPD) which is presumably an hereditary abnormality. The usual form of SPD involves an abnormality of the dense granules alone, which are either absent or upon platelet activation are unable to release locally their granule content (ATP, ADP, and serotonin). Another subgroup also has a defect in α-granule release products (factor VIII:vWF, platelet factor 4, β-thromboglobulin) as well. The diagnostic aggregation and nucleotide release patterns are as shown in this patient. The diagnosis can be confirmed by platelet electron microscopy, dense granule serotonin uptake and release and the measurement of α-granule release products.

There is no curative treatment but platelet transfusions will temporarily correct the bleeding tendency to cover any operative procedures. There is recent evidence that an infusion of DDAVP may also correct the bleeding time in some patients with SPD.

Long Case Answer 2

Further information required would be the blood group of the donor. Further investigations should include the testing of an eluate prepared from the patient's cells. This showed the presence of anti-A, and anti-B. The kidney donor was group O Rh Positive and 'passenger' B-lymphocytes in the transplanted kidney continued to produce anti-A and anti-B which react with the patients group A cells and the group A units cross-matched.

The patient was transfused group O cells without reaction.

Long Case Answer 3

This young girl clearly has acute lymphoblastic leukaemia. The marker studies show that this is of the common ALL variety (CALLA + DR + surface Ig −). The cells expressing T-cell antigens are the normal T cells — note that lymphocytes account for approximately 40% of the mononuclear cells in the blood.

CALLA positive ALL has a better prognosis than T, B, or 'null' ALL, but this girl can already be defined as being in a good prognostic group on the criteria of female sex, age between 2 and 12 years, and white cell count $< 20 \times 10^9/l$. The markers add little to the prognostic information.

Long Case Answer 4

This girl, who has had repeated red cell transfusions, has a condition resulting in either a shortened red cell survival, or a failure of production of red cells. One of the thalassaemic syndromes or sickle-thalassaemia are possible diagnoses. However, these are unlikely as she has no hepatosplenomegaly, normal facies, and relatively normal stature. There is no history of sickle pain crises as might be expected in sickle-thalassaemia. In β-thalassaemia major, hepatosplenomegaly is almost invariable, and there is usually hypertrophy of the facial bones due to erythroid hyperplasia. α-thalassaemia major with a four-gene deletion is incompatible with life, and with a three-gene deletion does not usually result in such severe anaemia. In addition she has a normal to raised mean cell volume with a low red cell count which would be unusual in β-thalassaemia major unless hypertransfused. Acute leukaemia or other haematological malignancy is unlikely as this child has had the disease all her life. Pure red cell aplasia is a possibility as she has a normal white cell count and platelet count and a borderline high MCV.

Examination of a blood film should be performed, with haemoglobin electrophoresis and a bone marrow examination. The latter will show increased erythroid activity with dyserythropoiesis in thalassaemias, or absence of erythroid activity in pure red cell aplasia. The ^{59}Fe counting data shown is typical of erythroid hypoplasia with decreased marrow uptake of iron and decreased incorporation into red cells. This child therefore has pure red cell aplasia of congenital kind (Blackfan-Diamond anaemia).

Long Case Answer 5

The likely diagnosis in this case is HbH disease. The red cells are microcytic, there is no iron deficiency and the haemoglobin electrophoresis shows a fast band (HbH) and a low A_2. The presence of 1% HbF is compatible with normal pregnancy.

The MCV of 72 fl is not as low as commonly found in HbH disease and is due to folic acid deficiency exacerbated by pregnancy. There is no evidence of B_{12} deficiency as B_{12} serum levels tend to be low in pregnancy.

This patient needs folate supplements and this may increase the haemoglobin a little. Transfusion is not indicated at this level of haemoglobin unless the fetus fails to grow satisfactorily, but the blood count should be monitored carefully. Any infections should be treated vigorously as this may cause marked falls in the haemoglobin. The disorder and its implications should be explained to the patient and her partner and the blood count (particularly the MCV) should be examined in the latter. If α-thalassaemia trait is suspected in the partner this should be confirmed by globin chain synthesis studies. The fetus can then be monitored by regular ultrasound examination to detect hydrops foetalis.

Long Case Answer 6

At diagnosis this woman had typical chronic lymphocytic leukaemia (CLL). The anaemia, raised MCV and reticulocytosis suggested the presence of immune haemolysis and this was confirmed by the finding of a positive direct antiglobulin test.

The likely cause of her acute abdomen is Richter's syndrome. This occurs in up to 5% of of cases of CLL, commonly as a pre-terminal event. A clone of cells expressing similar membrane phenotype to the original CLL cells arises and produces an invasive, rapidly growing tumour which often involves the para-aortic nodes. The tumour cells are usually very pleomorphic and multinucleate cells may be present.

Richter's-type transformation is very resistant to chemotherapy and, in view of her age, palliative therapy only is probably indicated. In a younger patient consideration should be given to a trial of combination chemotherapy such as CHOP.

Long Case Answer 7

1. The red cell mass of 1.9 litres represents a red cell mass of 40 ml/kg, which is well above the normal range for females (20–30 ml/kg). This confirms the polycythaemia suggested on the blood count. In view of the splenomegaly and raised white cell count a diagnosis of polycythaemia rubra vera can be made providing the arterial oxygen saturation is normal.
2. This woman now has severe anaemia, thrombocytopenia and marked splenomegaly, suggesting a myelofibrotic transformation of polycythaemia rubra vera. ^{59}Fe studies show little evidence of active erythropoiesis with no

uptake by the sacrum and little incorporation into the blood.

^{51}Cr surface counting shows progressive uptake by the spleen with regard to the liver. The actual counts and expected counts are shown in the table below:

Time	*Spleen*	*Liver*	*Heart*
Day 0	825	1000	760
Day 6 actual	1070	950	590
Day 6 expected (Day 0 × 590/760)	640	776	—
Excess Day 6 counts	430	174	—

Ratio of adjusted excess spleen to liver counts on Day 6 = 2.5

This result confirms the presence of hypersplenism but the decision to perform splenectomy was mainly dictated by her severe disomfort. Splenectomy resolved her abdominal symptoms and improved her blood count.

3. The disease has now progressed to a leukaemic phase with increased numbers of blast cells. Intensive anti-leukaemic therapy may be tried, but the disease is usually resistant, and in view of her age (66 years) palliative therapy with transfusions and hydroxyurea might be more appropriate.

Long Case Answer 8

The main problem is to decide whether the blood film changes are reactive or a primary phenomenon. The patient has a pleural effusion and despite a negative biopsy the possiblity of malignancy should be borne in mind. He has had two possible thromboembolic events which may be related to the high platelet count, either as cause or effect. Splenectomy is commonly associated with leucocytosis and thrombocytosis in the early postoperative period, and thereafter in the face of acute inflammatory or other events. On the other hand the platelet count and white cell count rather high to accept as reactive, particularly if they are a persistent phenomenon and if abnormal forms are present. Investigations which should help include marrow aspirate and trephine including chromosome analysis, neutrophil alkaline phosphatase score, and serum B_{12} and uric acid level. Clinical features such as haemorrhagic phenomenon, visual disturbance, microvascular occlusive symptoms or pruritus would suggest a primary myeloproliferative disorder. (The patient's marrow showed gross excess of normal megakaryocytes, abnormal myelopoiesis, and loss of sex chromosomes. A diagnosis of primary thrombocythaemia was made.)

Long Case Answer 9

Pre-operatively this man's coagulation was within normal limits. Immediately postoperatively there was a mild anaemia and thrombocytopenia which is usual following cardiac bypass surgery due to the dilutional effect of the banked blood and intravenous fluids used during the procedure in the pump circuits and to replace blood loss. The thrombin time and APTT were also slightly prolonged, which probably implies a combination of incomplete heparin reversal and dilution of the clotting factors during the operation. However, these minor degrees of haemostatic abnormality would not usually cause excessive postoperative bleeding. Six hours later the thrombin time and APTT were grossly prolonged although the platelet count was virtually unchanged and the prothrombin time was normal. The thrombin time corrected with protamine sulphate which specifically neutralises heparin, indicating the presence of circulating heparin as being responsible for the prolonged coagulation tests and the clinical bleeding problem. If heparin is incompletely neutralised after cardiac bypass surgery a so-called rebound phenomenon can occur 3–6 hours later with reappearance of significant amounts of heparin in the circulation, probably from the extravascular compartment. This can be rapidly corrected by a slow intravenous infusion of protamine sulphate. Other causes of bleeding following cardiac surgery which must be excluded include acute disseminated intravascular coagulation, generalised coagulation factor deficiency and/or thrombocytopenia due to massive transfusion, primary fibrinolysis and poor anatomical surgical stasis.

Long Case Answer 10

The clotting screen on this newborn baby showed a grossly prolonged prothrombin time and APTT but a thrombin time which, although slightly prolonged above the normal range, is the result that would be expected allowing for the liver immaturity of a full term neonate. These results suggest a deficiency of factor II, V and/or X which is not due to vitamin K deficiency. Isolated factor VII deficiency is excluded by a prolonged APTT and Stypven time. The Stypven time is dependent on direct activation of factor X by Russell's viper venom, thus bypassing factor VII activity. With isolated factor VII deficiency the Stypven time is normal. To determine which factor is deficient specific factor assays should be performed. However, if these are unavailable, correction tests on a prolonged prothrombin time can be helpful. Normal plasma, which contains all the coagulation factors, and normal serum, which contains factor V activity, caused a significant correction of the prolonged prothrombin time, thus excluding factor V deficiency. Plasma that has been adsorbed with aluminium hydroxide is specifically deficient in factors II, VII, IX and X. This only partially corrected the prolonged prothrombin time. This supports a diagnosis of factor II or X deficiency. Specific assays revealed an isolated factor X deficiency with an assay value of approximately 1% (normal 50–200%).

This child had severe congenital factor X deficiency which is inherited as an autosomal recessive condition. Bleeding episodes could be controlled by regular infusions of prothrombin complex concentrate (factor II, IX and X concentrate) or fresh frozen plasma.

Long Case Answer 11

This woman has a long history of thrombotic episodes and several related medical conditions which could be associated. When investigating a patient with a thrombotic disorder it is important to exclude a primary abnormality in the haemostatic mechanism (either congenital or acquired) which may predispose to such a condition. Secondarily one must determine whether there is a generalised hypercoagulable state involving the platelets, coagulation and fibrinolytic systems which may be exacerbating the thrombotic tendency. In this patient there is a grossly prolonged (virtually unclottable) thrombin time and a slightly prolonged APTT which fully corrects with 50% normal plasma (excluding a coagulation inhibitor). The possible causes of a prolonged thrombin time are a low fibrinogen level (hypofibrinogenaemia), an abnormal fibrinogen molecule (dysfibrinogenaemia), raised levels of fibrin(ogen) degradation products (FDPs) or the presence of heparin in the sample.

The failure of protamine sulphate to correct the prolonged thrombin time excludes the presence of heparin. The reptilase time is specifically prolonged in patients with a low or abnormal fibrinogen, and prolongation in this case suggests a fibrinogen defect. Quantitation of the fibrinogen molecule by two functional tests (clot weight and Clauss) and an immunological assay all revealed decreased levels from the normal range of 1.5–4 g/l. The functional assays were consistently lower than the immunological level suggesting the presence of a functionally abnormal molecule as well as hypofibrinogenaemia. Acquired abnormalities of the fibrinogen molecule do occur in patients with chronic liver disease and primary hepatoma, but this would seem highly unlikely in the presence of normal liver function tests. With the long history it is highly probable that the fibrinogen defect is hereditary. Certain dysfibrinogenaemias do predispose to repeated venous thrombosis and this is the most likely diagnosis in this patient.

Other specific congenital disorders which predispose to repeated thromboses and should be excluded are antithrombin III, protein C and protein S deficiency.

Long Case Answer 12

The initial coagulation screen shows a grossly prolonged bleeding time and a prolonged APTT which does not correct when incubated with 50% normal plasma. The factor VIII parameters show reduced VIII : C activity but virtually absent VIII : vWFag and VIII : vWF activity. Factor VIII : vWF is the biological functional assay of the von Willebrand's protein and is usually measured by the ristocetin co-factor assay. This assay determines the ability of patient's plasma to agglutinate formalin-fixed normal platelets in the presence of ristocetin and is dependent on large molecular weight multimers of von Willebrand's protein binding to glycoprotein Ib receptors on the platelet membrane surface. Factor VIII : vWFag (factor VIII : Rag by the old nomenclature) is the total antigenic activity of von Willebrand's protein determined by one of several immunological assays. In conclusion, this patients would appear to have a severe form of von Willebrand's disease. It is unusual for such a severe bleeding diathesis to present in later life and one would expect that this may be an acquired form. Indeed, there was no family history of bleeding problems and the patient had had a laparotomy some years before without postoperative bleeding.

Following an infusion of cryoprecipitate there was only a partial shortening of the APTT and bleeding time. Only factor VIII : C of the factor VIII parameters showed a significant increase. This poor response, particularly of the bleeding time and von Willebrand parameters, suggests the presence of an inhibitor (an acquired auto-antibody) to the von Willebrand protein. An inhibitor assay for factor VIII : C activity was negative and an appreciable rise in factor VIII : C levels occurred post-cryoprecipitate suggesting that the inhibitor was specific to the von Willebrand part of the molecule. A further inhibitor assay using the ristocetin co-factor technique confirmed the presence of a specific inhibitor.

The immediate short-term management to control severe and prolonged postoperative bleeding in a patient with acquired von Willebrand's disease is difficult and should only be undertaken in a specialist centre. Regular infusions of cryoprecipitate at 6–8 hourly intervals to control clinical bleeding should be given. The bleeding time, APTT, factor VIII : C and factor VIII : vWF should be monitored. If large volumes of cryoprecipitate are infused over several days there will be a persistent rise in the fibrinogen level, and a hyperviscosity-type syndrome may result if the level rises above 8 g/l. Unfortunately heat-treated factor VIII concentrates are unsuitable because they only contain VIII : C activity as VIII : vWF activity is destroyed by the preparatory fractionation process. In conjunction with cryoprecipitate infusions plasma exchange may assist in temporarily reducing the inhibitor level. Immunosuppressive therapy with azathioprine or cyclophosphamide is generally unhelpful in these cases.

Acquired von Willebrand's inhibitor may be associated with a paraprotein or lymphoma; these should be sought and the relevant treatment given if appropriate.

Long Case Answer 13

1. Autotransfusion is only recommended for patients with a normal haemoglobin ($>$ 11.5 g/dl in females).
2. Investigations should be directed at finding and treating the cause of her anaemia and identifying her atypical red cell antibodies.

   The serum ferritin may be falsely elevated in active collagen diseases, as it behaves as an acute phase protein. The high ESR in this case suggests that the rheumatoid disease is active. The serum iron and TIBC may be reduced in anaemia of chronic disease. To elucidate the cause of her anemia a bone marrow aspirate was performed. This showed absent iron stores, supporting a diagnosis of iron deficiency, possibly secondary to chronic gastrointestinal blood loss associated with NSAID treatment. After a month's treatment with oral iron the blood count showed WBC 7.0 $\times 10^9$/l, RBC 3.69 $\times 10^{12}$/l, Hb 9.1 g/dl, Hct .281, MCV 77 fl, MCH 24.7 pg, MCHC 32.4 g/dl.
3. Autotransfusion is still not possible as the haemoglobin is still too low, probably because of anaemia of chronic disease. The selection of units of donor blood negative for the public antigens Yk^a and Kn^a is logistically impossible. Public antigens, by definition, are present on the red cells of more than 90% of unselected donors.
4. The survival curve shows a red cell half-life of approximately 22 days (normal 25 days). This is estimated by finding the point on the graph corresponding to 50% survival on the vertical axis and

reading off the corresponding time in days on the horizontal axis. Although the survival time of these units is not normal, it would not be expected that SAG-M stored red cells would have a completely normal survival time.

The hip replacement operation was performed with six units of v negative blood being transfused. There was no reaction, and the postoperative haemoglobin was 13.8 g/dl.

Long Case Answer 14

1. This patient has a normochromic anaemia and mild leucopenia. The blood film shows markedly abnormal red cells with gross anisocytosis, and neutrophil hypersegmentation. Occasional tear drop shaped macrocytes are present. The bone marrow aspirate demonstrates megaloblastic erythropoiesis. Iron stain was performed on another slide, which showed normal iron stores, without sideroblastic change.
2. The haematological diagnosis is megaloblastic anaemia secondary to vitamin B_{12} deficiency in a patient with β-thalassaemia trait.
3. In view of the weight loss, abdominal symptoms and the patient's normal diet, malabsorption of B_{12} seems likely. A Schilling test should therefore be performed.
4. The Schilling test demonstrates intestinal malabsorption of B_{12}. This should be investigated by barium studies, faecal fat estimation or vitamin A absorption test, duodenal or jejunal biopsies, and stool and gastric juice examination for Giardia and other parasites.

   This patient was found to have Crohn's disease affecting the terminal ileum. His megaloblastic anaemia responded well to vitamin B_{12} and his MCV and MCH dropped to thalassaemic levels as the haemoglobin rose.

FURTHER READING

Long Case 1

Holmsen H, Weiss H J 1972 Further evidence for a deficient storage pool of adenine nucleotides in platelets from some patients with thrombocytopathis — 'storage pool disease'. Blood 39: 197

Long Case 2

Bevan P C, Seaman Muriel, Tolliday B, Chalmers D G 1985 ABO haemolytic anaemia in transplanted patients. Vox Sanguinis 49: 42

Long Case 3

Bloomfield C D 1981 Classification and prognosis of acute lymphoblastic leukaemia. Prognostic Clinical and Biological Research 58: 167

Robinson L L, Nesbit M E, Sather H N, Hammond G D, Coccia P F 1980 Assessment of the interrelationship of prognostic factors in childhood acute lymphoblastic leukaemia. A report from Children's Cancer Study Group. American Journal of Pediatric Hematology Oncology 2: 5

Long Case 4

Alter B P 1980 Childhood red cell aplasia. American Journal of Pediatric Hematology and Oncology 2: 121

Finch C A et al 1970 Ferrokinetics in man. Medicine 49: 17

Long Case 5

Weatherall D J, Clegg J B 1980 The thalassaemia syndromes, 3rd edn. Blackwell Scientific Publications, Oxford

Long Case 6

Foucan K, Rydell R E 1980 Richter's syndrome in chronic lymphocytic leukaemia. Cancer 46: 118

Long Case 7

Benbassat J, Penchas S, Ligumski M 1979 Splenectomy in patients with agnogenic myeloid metaplasia: an analysis of 321 reported cases. British Journal of Haematology 42: 207

Wasserman L R 1954 Polycythaemia vera — its course and treatment: relation to myeloid metaplasia and leukaemia. Bulletin of the New York Academy of Medicine 3: 343

Long Case 8

Gunz F W 1960 Hemorrhagic thrombocythaemia: a critical review. Blood 15: 706

Hardisty R M, Wolff H H 1955 Haemorrhagic thrombocythaemia: a clinical and laboratory study. British Journal of Haematology 1: 390

Long Case 9

Salzman E W, Deykin D, Shapiro R M, Rosenberg R 1975 Management of heparin therapy: controlled prospective trial. New England Journal of Medicine 292: 1046

Long Case 10

Denson K W E, Lurie A, de Cataldo P, Mannucci P M 1970 The factor X defect: recognition of abnormal forms of factor X. British Journal of Haematology 18: 317

Long Case 11

D'Souza L, Coots M C, Glueck H I 1979 An acquired abnormal fibrinogen associated with thromboembolic disease and pseudotumor cerebri. Thrombosis Haemostasis 42: 994

Long Case 12

Ingram C I C, Kingston P J, Leslie J, Bowie E J W 1971 Four cases of acquired von Willebrand's syndrome. British Journal of Haematology

Long Case 13

Kay L M 1987 The need for autologous blood transfusion. British Medical Journal 294: 137

Mollison P L, Engelfriet C P, Contraras M 1988 Blood transfusion in clinical medicine, 8th edn. Blackwell, Oxford, p 406

Long Case 14

Steinberg F 1961 The megaloblastic anaemia of regional ileitis. New England Journal of Medicine 264: 186

5 MRCP Slide Questions

Slide 5.1

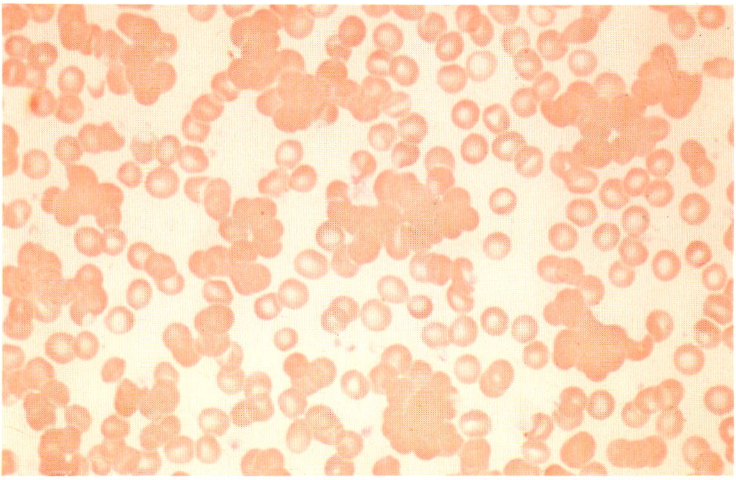

A 74-year-old woman attended her GP complaining of Raynaud's phenomenon, which she had read about in a magazine. Physical examination was normal except for a discoloured nose. He performed a blood count: WBC 7.5 $\times$ 10^9/l, RBC 3.07 $\times$ 10^{12}/l, Hb 14.5 g/dl, PCV 32.2, MCV 104.9 fl, MCH 47.2 pg, MCHC 45.1 g/dl, platelets 217 $\times$ 10^9/l. Differential: neutrophils 29%, lymphocytes 65%, monocytes 5%, eosinophils 1%.
The blood film is shown above.

1. What is the likely cause of her Raynaud's phenomenon?
2. What is the possible cause of the blood count abnormalities?
3. What further investigations should be performed?
4. What is the treatment?

Slide 5.2

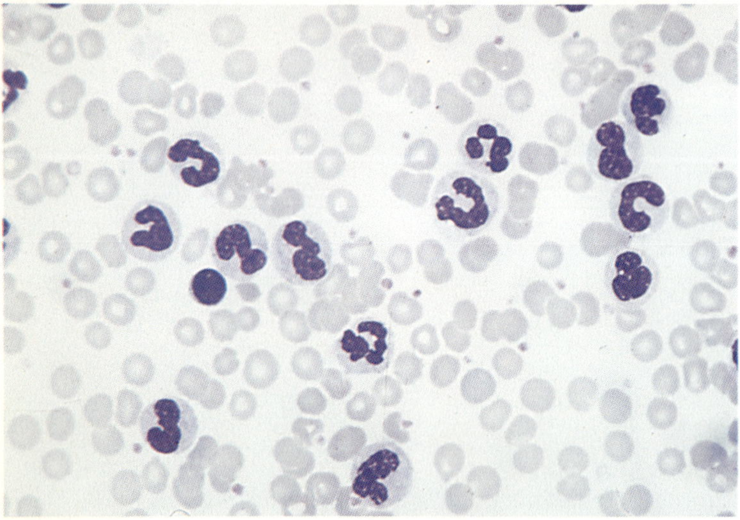

The slide above shows the peripheral blood film from a 63-year-old man who presented with a perforated peptic ulcer. Haemoglobin 13.0 g/l, WBC 87.6×10^9/l, platelets 400 $\times 10^9$/l.

1. What two haematological conditions are possible?
2. Give two investigations and one clinical sign that will establish the haematological diagnosis.
3. What is the natural history of this condition?

Slide 5.3

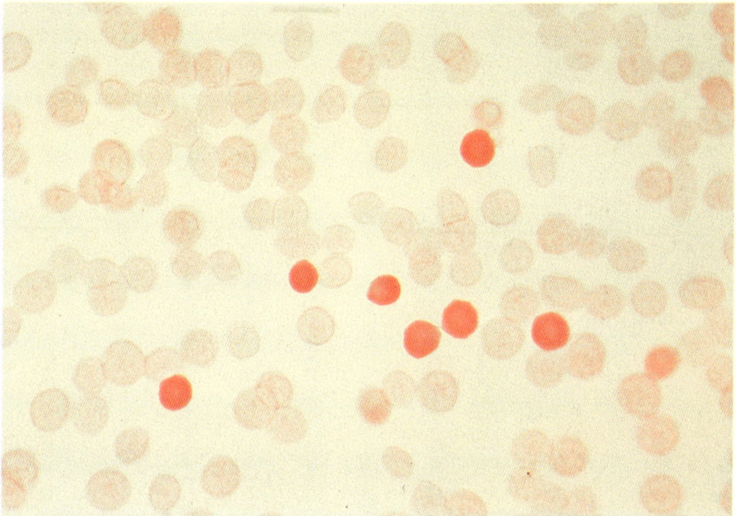

A 3.5 kg full term baby was noted to be pale, but not jaundiced, at delivery. Blood count showed a haemoglobin of 11.2 g/dl. A maternal blood sample stained by the Kleihauer technique for fetal haemoglobin is shown above.

1. Comment on the appearances.
2. When is the Kleihauer test usually performed?
3. In what condition not associated with pregnancy is the Kleihauer test positive?

Slide 5.4

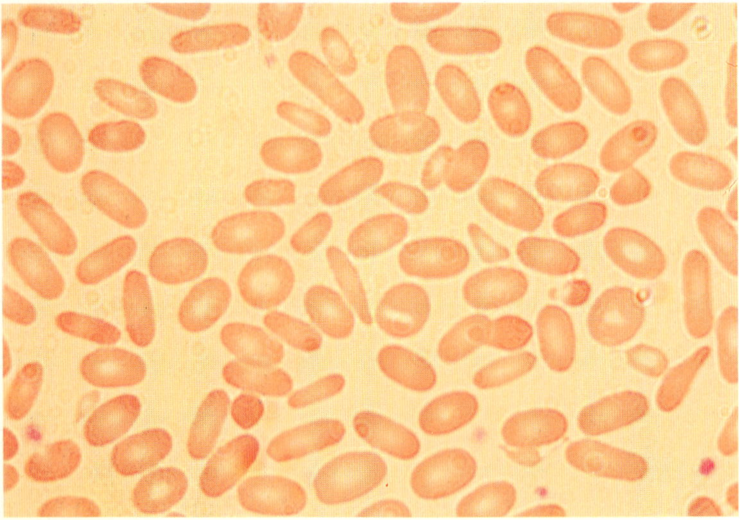

A 55-year-old man was admitted for repair of inguinal hernia. Routine pre-operative blood count was normal, but the blood film (shown above) was noted to be abnormal.

1. What abnormality is shown?
2. What treatment is required?
3. What is the relationship of this condition with the Rhesus blood groups?

Slide 5.5

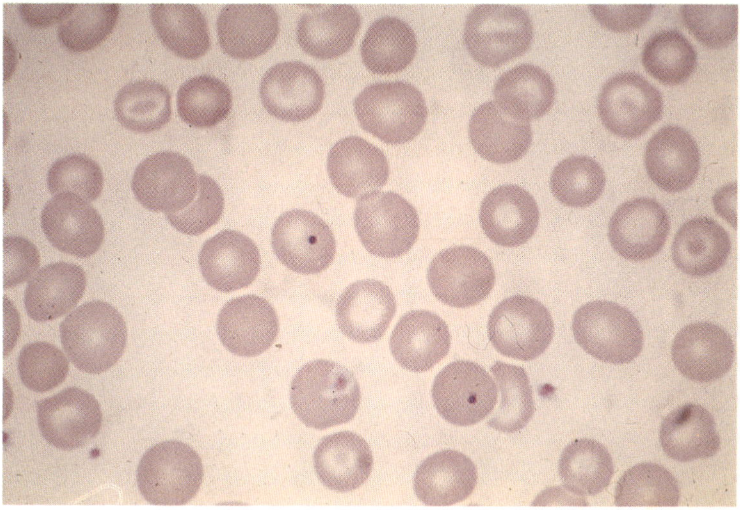

A 35-year-old woman is seen in the antenatal booking clinic. She gave a history of idiopathic thrombocytopenic purpura (ITP), though she had had no treatment for this for 15 years.

Blood count showed: WBC 11.1 × 10^9/l, Hb 11.3 g/dl, platelets 219 × 10^9/l, neutrophils 63%, lymphocytes 27%. The blood film is shown above.

1. State three abnormalities seen on the blood film.
2. What is their cause?
3. What advice should you give the obstetrician?

Slide 5.6

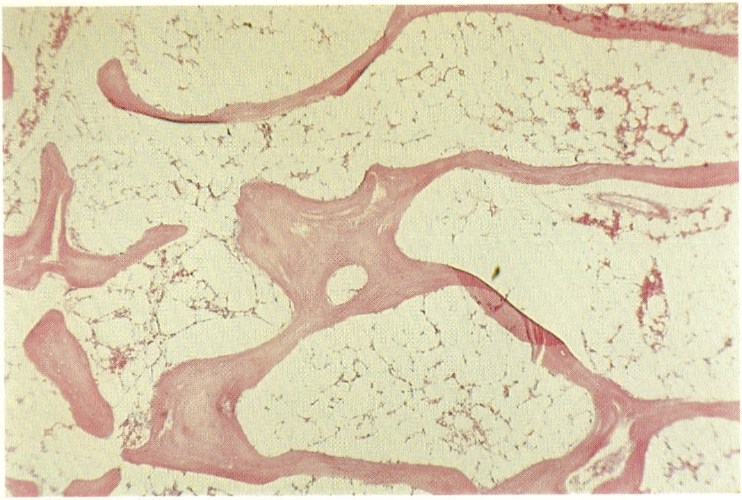

A 24-year-old man presented with a purpuric rash and weakness. Blood count showed: WBC 2.1 × 10^9/l, Hb 8.7 g/dl, platelets 23 × 10^9/l, neutrophils 23%, lymphocytes 73%, monocytes 2%. Bone marrow trephine biopsy is shown above.

1. What is the diagnosis?
2. What are the causes of this condition?
3. What marrow pathologies are best diagnosed by trephine as opposed to aspiration biopsy?

Slide 5.9

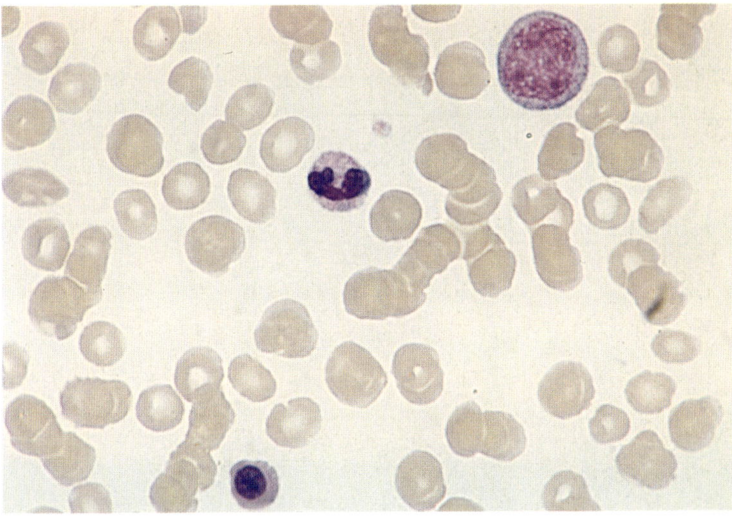

The blood film from a 63-year-old man with a right hilar mass on chest X-ray is shown above. The haemoglobin is 9.6 g/dl.

Comment on the blood film and give your conclusions.

Slide 5.10

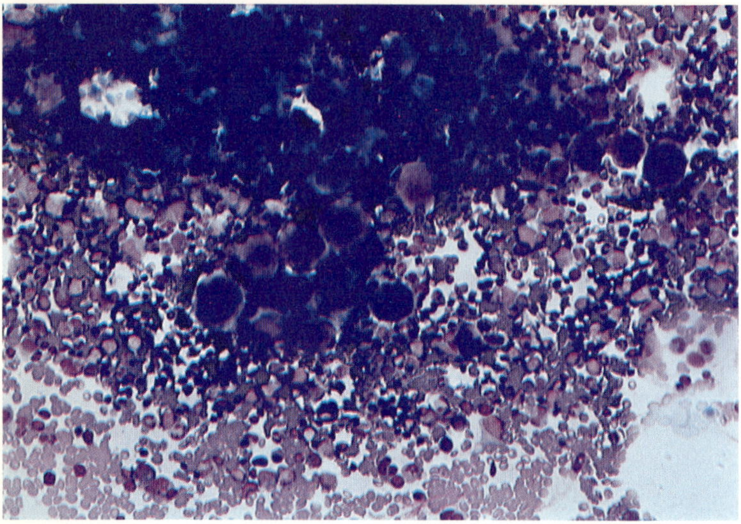

This is the bone marrow aspirate of a 5-year-old girl who developed nose bleeds and petechial rash following an upper respiratory tract infection. Hb 11.0 g/dl, WBC 10.5 $\times 10^9$/l, platelets 8 $\times 10^9$/l. Blood film shows a few reactive lymphocytes but otherwise normal white cells.

What is the likely diagnosis?

Slide 5.11

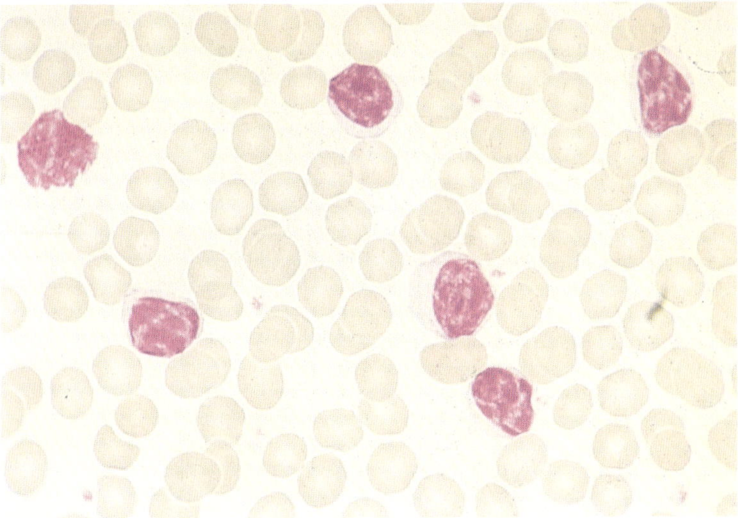

The blood film from a 72-year-old man admitted with a myocardial infarct is shown above. Hb 14.6 g/dl, WBC 42.0 $\times 10^9/l$, platelets 186 $\times 10^9/l$.

What is the diagnosis?

Slide 5.12

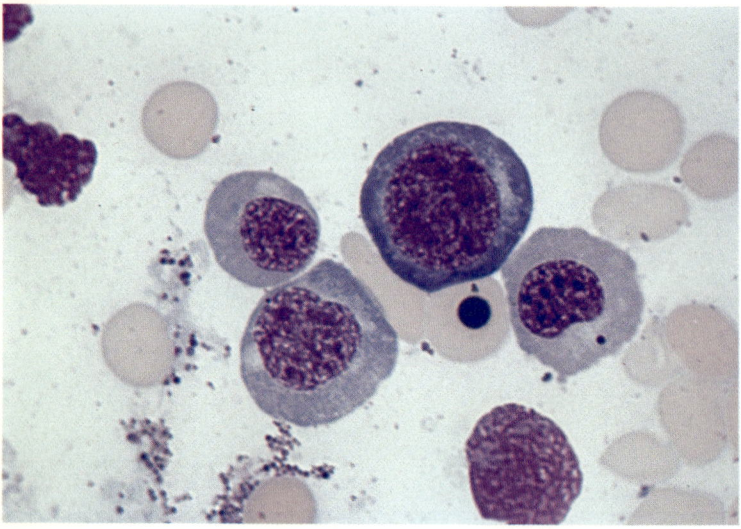

The slide above shows the bone marrow aspirate from a severely anaemic woman.

What features are shown?

Slide 5.13

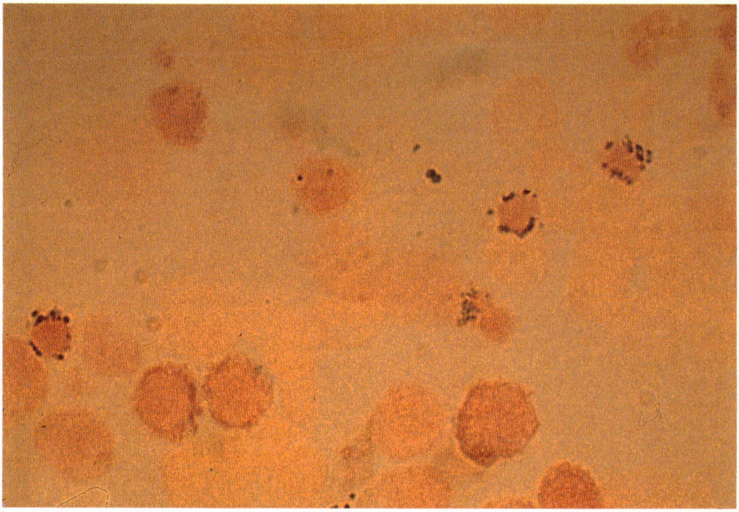

A bone marrow aspirate from a 65-year-old man being investigated for macrocytic anaemia is shown above. It has been stained by Perl's ferrocyanide reaction.

What abnormality is shown and what are its causes?

Slide 5.14

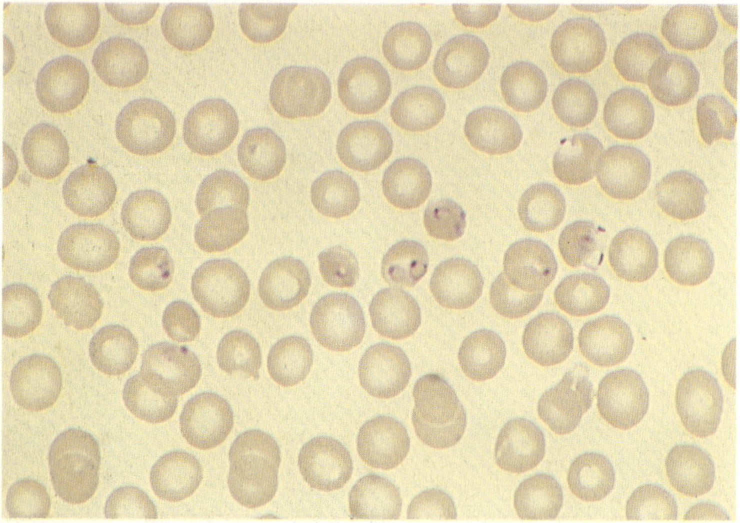

The blood film from a 19-year-old undergraduate is shown above. He had returned from a field trip to East Africa two days before.

What is the diagnosis?

Slide 5.15

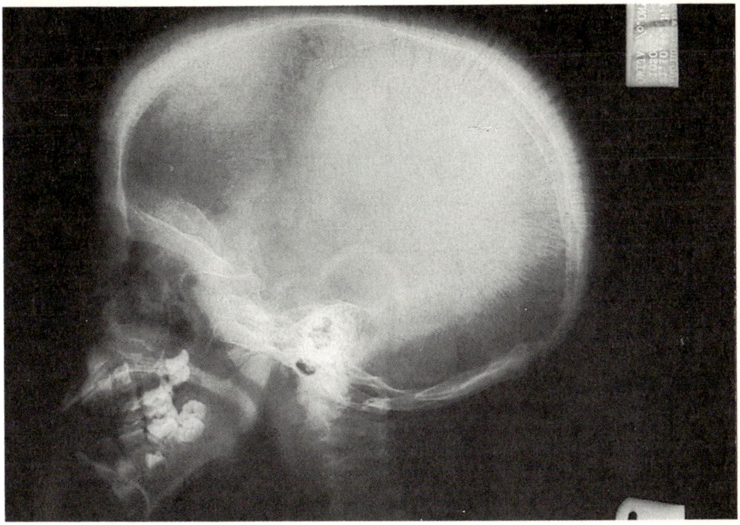

The lateral skull X-ray of a haematology patient is shown above.

What abnormality is shown?

Slide 5.16

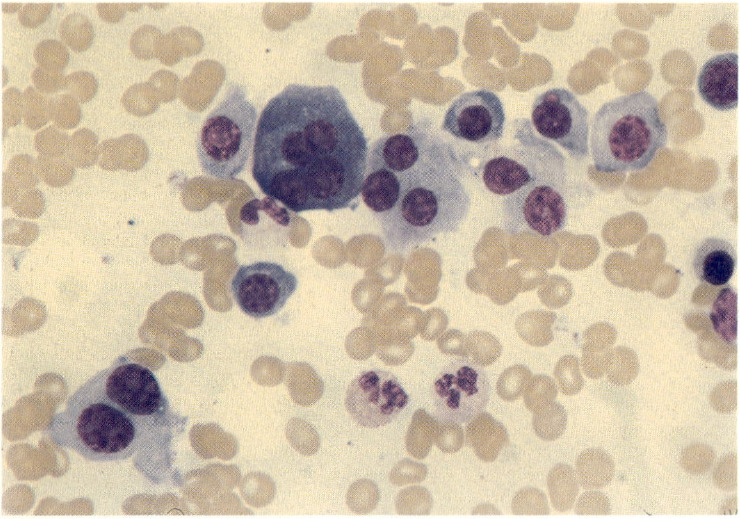

Bone marrow aspirate from a patient with a leucoerythroblastic anaemia is shown above.

What is the diagnosis?

Slide 5.17

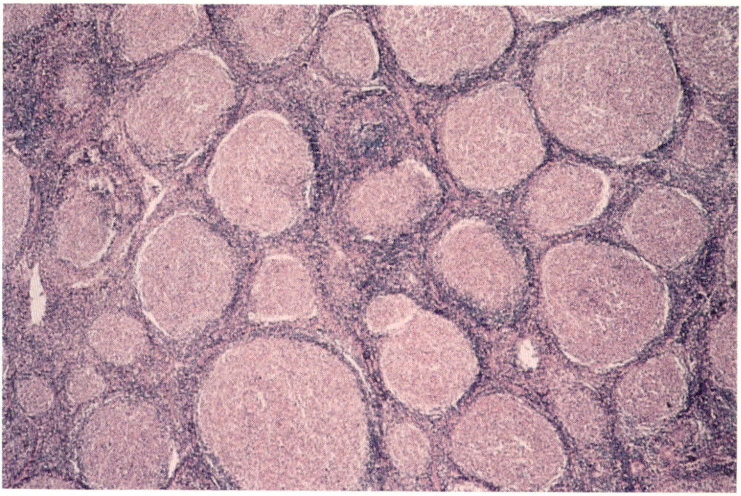

A 45-year-old patient presents with cervical lymphadenopathy. An enlarged lymph node is biopsied. An H&E stained section is shown above.

What is the diagnosis and prognosis?

Slide 5.18

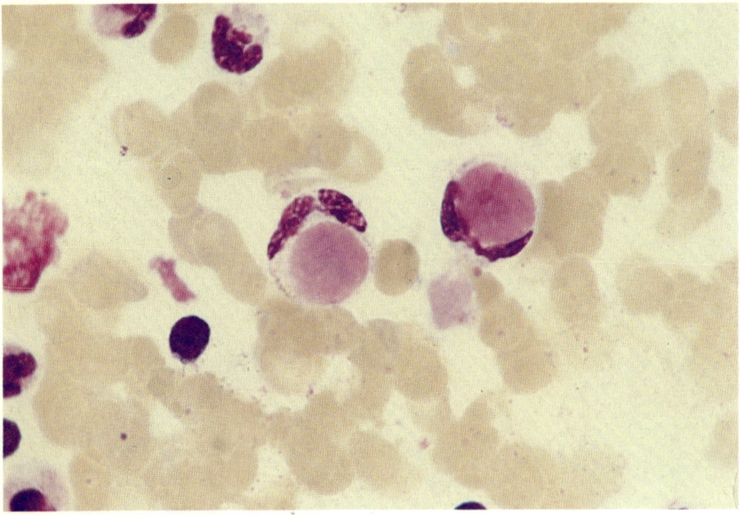

The spun deposit from a pleural effusion is shown above.

What phenomenon is shown?

Slide 5.19

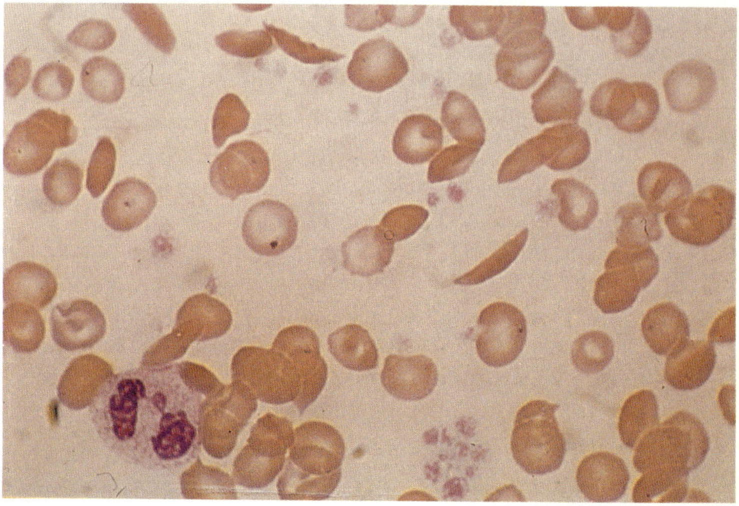

The peripheral blood from an anaemic patient is shown above.

What abnormalities are shown and what is the diagnosis?

Answers/Comments

Slide 5.1

The blood film shows cold agglutinates. These are haphazard clumps of red cells agglutinated by an auto-antibody in her serum. This works at temperatures below 37°C — a 'cold' antibody. When her hands get cold, symptoms of microvascular occlusion by agglutinates occur.

The blood count demonstrates nonsense indices caused by the blood cell counter counting clumps of red cells rather than single red cells. The red cell agglutinates were only partially dispersed by warming the sample to 37°C before processing.

The blood count also demonstrates a lymphocytosis. Cold agglutinins may be a manifestation of underlying lymphoma. Bone marrow, protein electrophoresis, immunoglobulins, and radiological investigation of chest and abdomen to look for enlarged lymph nodes should be performed.

The mainstay of treatment for cold agglutinin disease is keeping the patient WARM. Steroids and splenectomy tend to be less effective than in warm auto-immune haemolytic anaemia, but chlorambucil may be useful. Folic acid is administered as in any cause of haemolysis.

Other causes of Raynaud's phenomenon are cryoglobulins. (i.e. a globulin protein that precipitates in the cold, not having known antibody specificity), cervical rib, scleroderma, and ingestion of vasoconstrictors.

Slide 5.2

The film shows large numbers of neutrophils, compatible with the very high white cell count. This is a neutrophil leukaemoid reaction. The other possibility is chronic granulocytic leukaemia (CGL) but the type of granulocytes on the film make this unlikely — in CGL, the white cell differential shows many (up to 40%) immature granulocytes, particularly myelocytes but also metamyelocytes, promyelocytes and a few myeloblasts. The neutrophils in a leukaemoid reaction are usually mature cells, perhaps with some left shift of nuclear maturation, and often show toxic granulation. A second useful discriminatory test is a special stain of a blood film to demonstrate neutrophil alkaline phosphatase (NAP). This will be high in a leukaemoid reaction but low, or even zero, in CGL. Although seldom necessary in a case such as this, chromosome analysis of bone marrow cells will be normal in a leukaemoid reaction, but will demonstrate the Philadelphia chromosome in most cases of CGL. A useful discriminatory physical sign is the presence of splenomegaly, usual in CGL but not seen in leukaemoid reactions. Leukaemoid reactions tend to subside rapidly as the underlying illness (commonly severe acute infection) comes under control. This patient's WBC was 14.0 $\times 10^9$/l six days later.

Slide 5.3

Numerous darkly stained fetal cells are seen against a background of pale staining maternal cells. The Kleihauer technique elutes adult haemoglobin from maternal cells using an acid buffer, whilst fetal haemoglobin is resistant to acid elution. In this case, quantitation performed by counting the ratio of fetal to maternal cells suggested a fetal–maternal bleed of 200 ml, causing a neonatal anaemia.

The Kleihauer fetal cell test is usually performed to measure fetal–maternal haemorrhage at delivery of a Rhesus positive baby to a Rhesus negative mother, in order to assess the need for further injections of anti-D.

People with hereditary persistence of fetal haemoglobin may have either diffusely or heterogeneously positive staining red cells in their blood.

Slide 5.4

The blood film shows numerous elliptocytes — red cells that are ellipsoidal in shape rather than round.

The majority of patients with this abnormality require no treatment as significant haemolysis is unusual. In the event of haemolysis occurring, the disorder is treated as for hereditary spherocytosis.

Inheritance is usually autosomal dominant, and linkage to the Rhesus blood group can often be demonstrated.

Slide 5.5

Target cells, Howell-Jolly bodies and a spherocyte. These changes are due to hyposplenism, in this case due to previous splenectomy for treatment of ITP. Other changes seen after splenectomy include a lower level of IgM in the serum, iron granules in the red cells, red cell poikilocytosis, a slight increase in reticulocyte count, and an enhanced leucocytosis in response to infection.

This patient is not at risk from bleeding at this platelet count, though her platelet count should be monitored as ITP may relapse during pregnancy. The baby's platelet count should also be measured, as passive antibody transfer from the mother may cause it to be thrombocytopenic.

Slide 5.6

The marrow shows gross hypocellularity — aplastic anaemia. Aplastic anaemia may be secondary to drug idiosyncrasy (e.g. gold, Butazolidin, chloramphenicol), radiation, or administration of cytotoxics. It may also be associated with viral hepatitis and paroxysmal nocturnal haemoglobinuria. The majority of cases presenting de novo are idiopathic, some of which are auto-immune in nature.

Marrow trephine biopsy is essential, being a more reliable method than aspirate in diagnosing secondary deposits, lymphoma, myelofibrosis; it will also be required when a dry tap is obtained on aspirate.

Slide 5.7

Patient X has two major bands on cellulose acetate electrophoresis, one in the region of HbA and one in the HbS region. A third minor, normal band in the HbA2/C region is also present. On agar gel electrophoresis at acid pH the strip is the same as the HbA/A control, with a major band in HbA region and a weak normal band representing HbF. The probable genotype is HbD trait. HbD moves with HbS at pH 9.2 but with HbA at pH 6.0. This variant is usually suspected when a band in the HbS region is identified on routine cellulose acetate electrophoresis, but the sickle cell solubility test is negative.

Slide 5.8

Oval macrocytes, hypersegmented polymorphs and cell fragments: megaloblastic anaemia.

Slide 5.9

Rouleaux, nucleated red cell and myelocyte present — a leucoerythroblastic blood film. In view of the clinical story a bronchial carcinoma with bone marrow metastases must be considered.

Slide 5.10

The marrow shows an increase in immature megakaryocytes, indicating that peripheral destruction of platelets is the cause of the thrombocytopenia. The child has immune thrombocytopenia, probably as a result of a recent viral infection.

Slide 5.11

Chronic lymphocytic leukaemia — all the cells present are mature-looking lymphocytes plus a smear cell. The latter are produced by damage to the fragile CLL lymphocytes during film preparation.

Slide 5.12

Megaloblastic erythroblasts at all stages of maturation. The major features of megaloblastic erythropoiesis are premature haemoglobinisation and chromatin deficiency. As the erythroblast matures it manufactures haemoglobin, which turns the cytoplasm from blue to pink. At the same time the nucleus shrinks, becomes pyknotic, and is extruded from the cell. These megaloblasts have haemoglobinised cytoplasm with relatively immature nuclei which have a lacy appearance — chromatin deficiency.

Slide 5.13

Perl's ferrocyanide reaction stains iron blue–green. This slide shows ringed sideroblasts — the pathognomonic feature of sideroblastic change. Developing erythroblasts frequently contain one or two iron granules in order to manufacture haemoglobin. In sideroblastic anaemia there is failure to incorporate iron into haemoglobin and it accumulates in the mitochondria which lie in a ring around the nucleus.

Sideroblastic change is seen in primary sideroblastic anaemia, and as a secondary phenomenon in the collagen diseases, alcoholism, in association with malignancy, heavy metal poisoning and during treatment with isoniazid, cycloserine and chloramphenicol.

Slide 5.14

Falciparum (malignant tertian) malaria. Multiple ring-form trophozoites are present in non-enlarged red cells.

Slide 5.15

Marrow expansion ('hair on end') appearance due to erythroid hyperplasia. This appearance may be seen in the congenital haemolytic anaemias — β-thalassaemia major and sickle cell anaemia. Prognathism (hyperplasia of the maxilla and mandible) is also a feature.

Slide 5.16

Multiple myeloma. All but two of the cells present are plasma cells, including atypical multinucleate forms. Normally up to 5% of nucleated cells in the bone marrow are plasma cells. Up to 20% plasma cells may be found as a reaction to chronic infection, malignancy or collagen disease. More than 20% plasma cells is virtually diagnostic of myeloma.

Slide 5.17

The lymph node is replaced by nodules of lymphoma — follicular lymphoma. The presence of a follicular rather than diffuse pattern of histology is associated with a good prognosis.

Slide 5.18

Two LE (lupus erythematosus) cells are shown. The LE cell is a neutrophil whose nucleus is displaced by an amorphous ingested lymphocyte nucleus. This phenomenon may be seen in effusions or (rarely) in the blood from patients with systemic lupus erythematosus. LE cells are also seen in the LE preparation. In this test blood is defibrinated or shaken with glass beads to damage the lymphocytes. It is then incubated so that neutrophils may ingest the exposed nuclear material in the presence of anti-nuclear antibodies. The LE cell test is relatively insensitive and laborious for the diagnosis of SLE. It has been replaced by tests for anti-nuclear antibodies.

Slide 5.19

Sickle cells, target cells and Howell-Jolly bodies. This patient has sickle cell anaemia. Auto-splenectomy due to repeated infarctions is usual in these patients, which explains the Howell-Jolly bodies.

FURTHER READING

Slide 5.1
MacKenzie M R, Fundenberg H H 1972 Macroglobulinaemia: an analysis of forty patients. Blood 39: 874
Slide 5.2
Hilts S V, Shaw C C 1953 Leukaemoid blood reactions. New England Journal of Medicine 249: 434

Slide 5.3
McLarey D C, Fish S A 1966 Fetal erythrocytes in the maternal circulation. American Journal of Obstetrics and Gynecology 95: 824
Slide 5.4
Bannerman R M, Renwick J H 1962 The hereditary elliptocytoses: clinical and linkage data. Annals of Human Genetics 26: 23
Slide 5.5
Ek J I, Rayner S 1950 An analytical study of splenectomised cases after traumatic rupture of the spleen. Acta Medica Scandinavia 137: 417
Laros R K Jr, Sweet R L 1975 Management of idiopathic thrombocytopenic purpura during pregnancy. American Journal of Obstetrics and Gynecology 122: 182
Slide 5.6
Thomas E D (ed) 1987 Aplastic anaemia. Clinics in Haematology 7
Slide 5.7
Dacie J V, Lewis S M 1984 Practical Haematology. Churchill Livingstone, Edinburgh, p 186
Slide 5.8
Lindenbaum J, Nath B J 1980 Megaloblastic anaemia and neutrophil hypersegmentation. British Journal of Haematology 44: 511
Slide 5.9
Weick J K, Hagedorn J B, Linman J W 1974 Leucoerythroblastosis: diagnostic and prognostic significance. Mayo Clinic Proceedings 49: 111
Slide 5.10
McWilliams N B, Mauer H M 1979 Acute idiopathic thrombocytopenia in children. American Journal of Hematology 7: 87
Slide 5.11
Hamblin T J 1987 Chronic lymphocytic leukaemia. Clinical Haematology 1(2): 449
Slide 5.12
Hoffbrand A V 1981 In: Hoffbrand A V, Lewis S M (eds) Megaloblastic anaemias in postgraduate haematology. William Heinemann, London, p 72.
Slide 5.13
Mollin D L 1965 Sideroblasts and sideroblastic anaemia. British Journal of Haematology 11: 41
Slide 5.14
Perrin L H, MacKey L J, Miesher P A 1982 The hematology of malaria in man. Seminars in Haematology 19: 70
Slide 5.15
Moseley J E 1963 Bone changes in hematological disorders (roentgen aspects). Grune and Stratton, New York
Slide 5.16
Drivsholm A, Clausen J 1964 The relationship between the cytology and the immunoelectrophoretic pattern in 105 cases of myelomatosis. Acta Medica Scandinavia 175: 609
Slide 5.17
Berard C W, Dorfman R F 1974 Histopathology of malignant lymphomas. Clinics in Haematology 3(1): 77
Slide 5.18
Koller S R, Johnston C L, Moncure C W, Waller M V 1976 Lupus erythematosus cell preparation — antinuclear factor incongruity. A review of diagnostic tests for systemic lupus erythematosus. American Journal of Clinical Pathology 66: 495
Slide 5.19
Fleming A F 1982 Sickle cell disease. Churchill Livingstone, Edinburgh

6 MRCPath Slide Questions

Slide 6.1

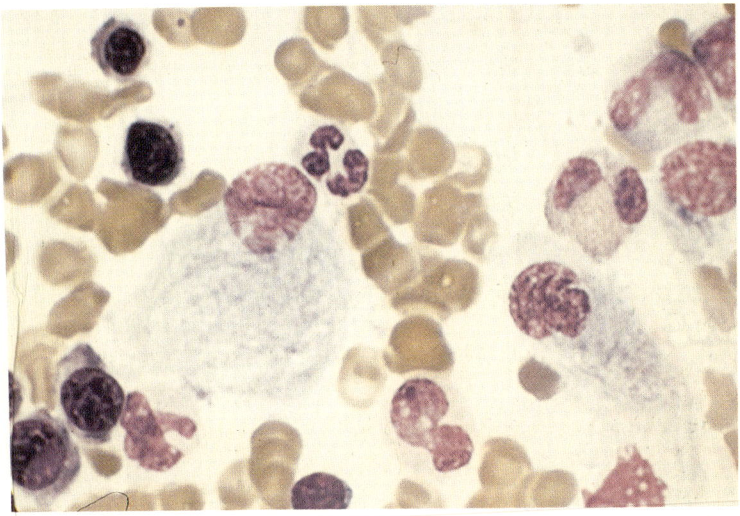

A 29-year-old man attended the chest clinic with a three-month history of chest pain radiating to the left shoulder. He gave a history of easy bruising for many years, and had bled for one hour after a tooth extraction two years before.

On examination the only abnormality was a 3 cm palpable spleen. Blood count showed: WBC 4.0 × 10^9/l, Hb 13.3 g/dl, platelets 95 × 10^9/l neutrophils 49%, lymphocytes 48%, monocytes 3%, ESR 25 mm/h.

Bone marrow aspirate examination was performed (shown above).

1. What is the diagnostic feature shown?
2. What was the cause of his pain?
3. What confirmatory diagnostic tests are available?

Slide 6.2

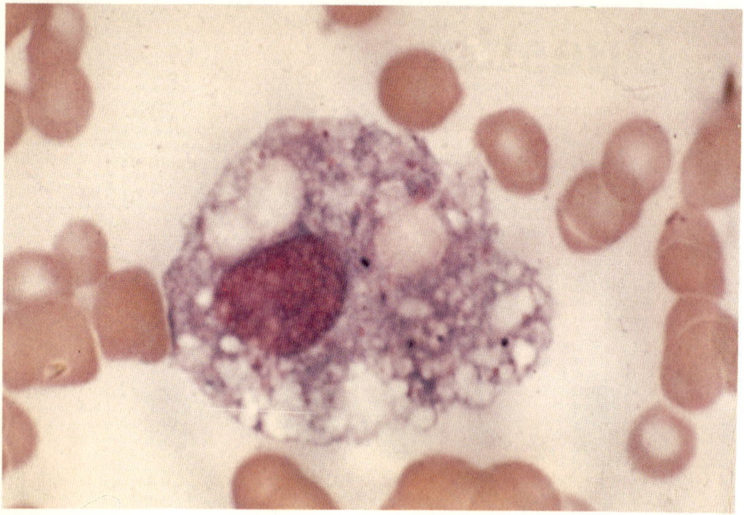

Bone marrow aspirate from a 40-year-old woman is shown above.

1. What is this cell?
2. What phenomenon is shown?
3. What are its causes?

Slide 6.3

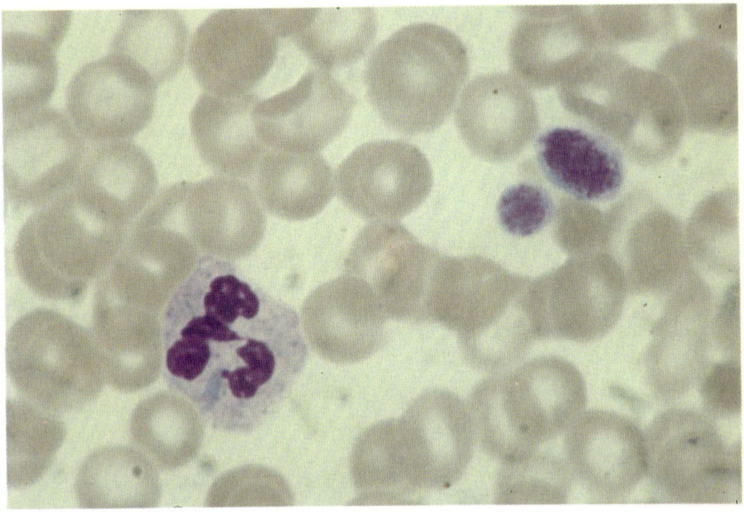

A blood film from a 21-year-old woman who presented with a mild thrombocytopenia (platelets $93 \times 10^9/l$) is shown above.

Comment on the morphology.

Slide 6.4

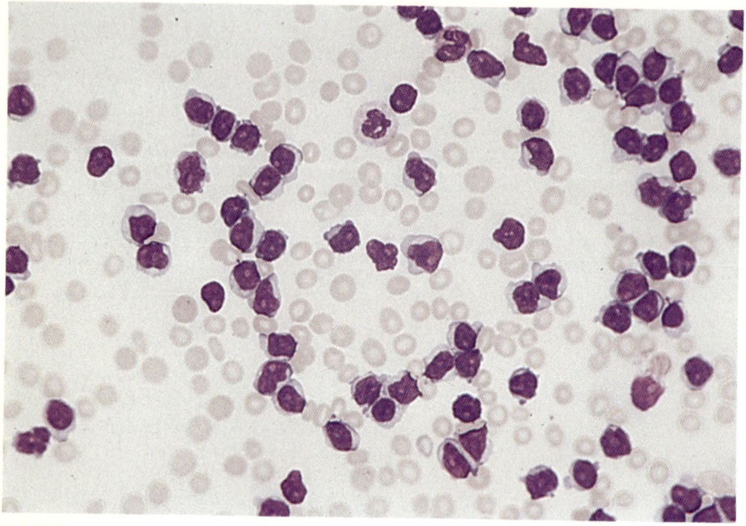

The blood film above is taken from a man of 73 who presented with general malaise and splenomegaly.

1. What is the likely diagnosis?
2. What surface marker characteristics would you expect?

Slide 6.5

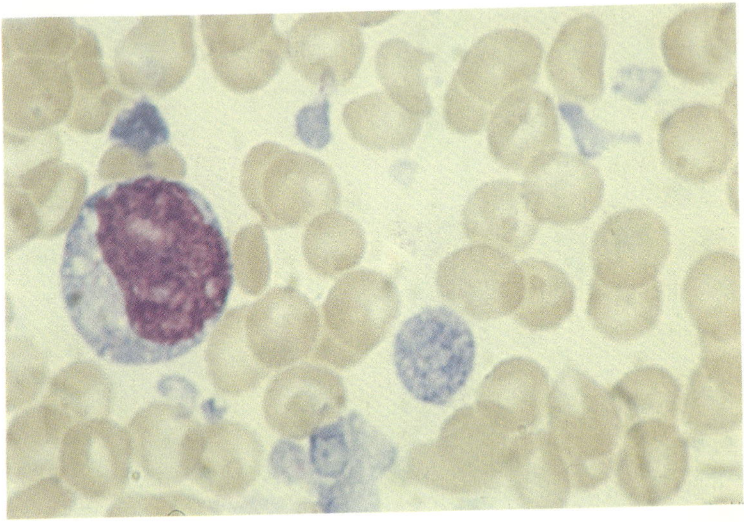

The blood film shown above was taken from a patient with acute leukaemia.

What abnormalities are shown?

Slide 6.6

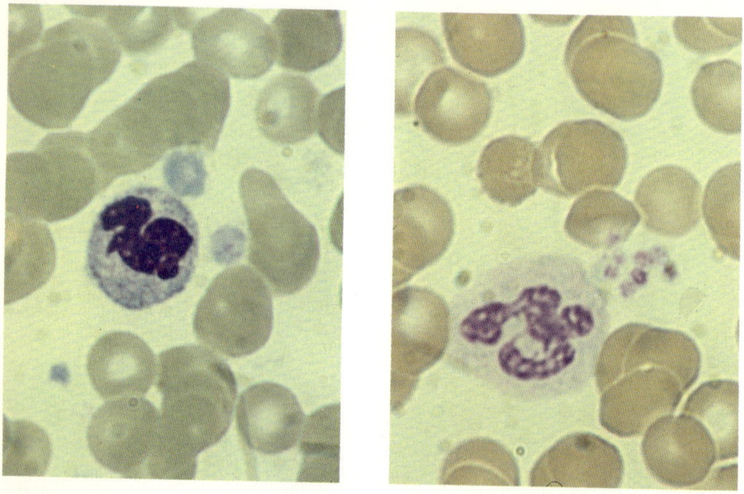

A 21-year-old woman presented with mild thrombocytopenia (platelet count 80 × $10^9/1$) and a mild bleeding tendency. Her blood film is shown above (left). For comparison, a normal blood film is shown on the right hand side.

Comment on the platelet morphology of the blood film.

Slide 6.7

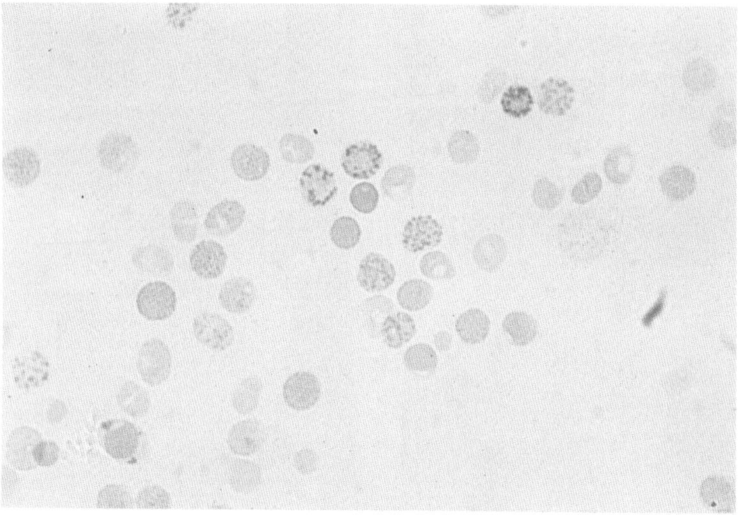

This is a reticulocyte preparation from a pregnant 20-year-old woman who has had moderate anaemia and splenomegaly since childhood. Hb is currently 8.0 g/dl.

What is the diagnosis?

Slide 6.8

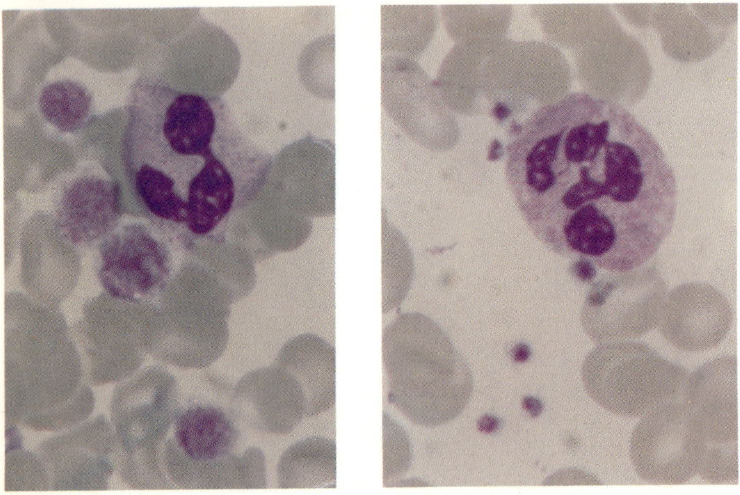

Comment on the platelet morphology of the blood film shown above left, from a 6-year-old boy who presented with excessive gum bleeding. For comparison, the blood film on the right, stained at the same time, is from a normal healthy adult.

Slide 6.9

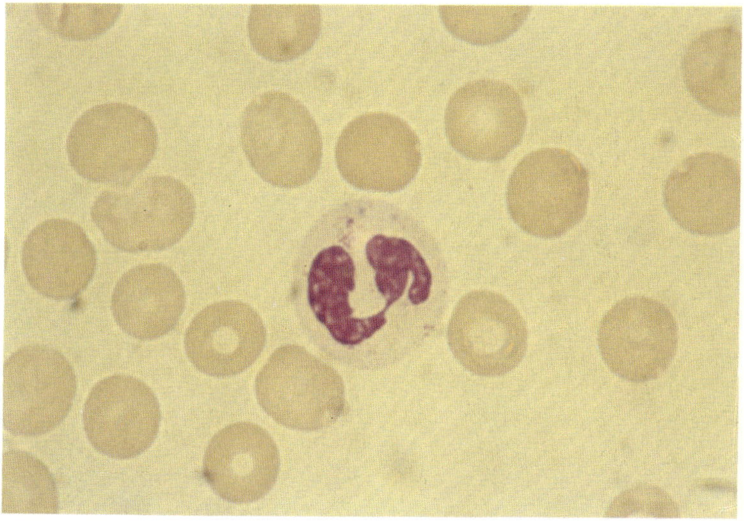

An elderly woman presented with recurrent chest infections, an extensive herpes simplex lesion on her lip and scattered petechial haemorrhages on her legs. This is her peripheral blood film.

What features are illustrated and what are the possible diagnoses?

Slide 6.10

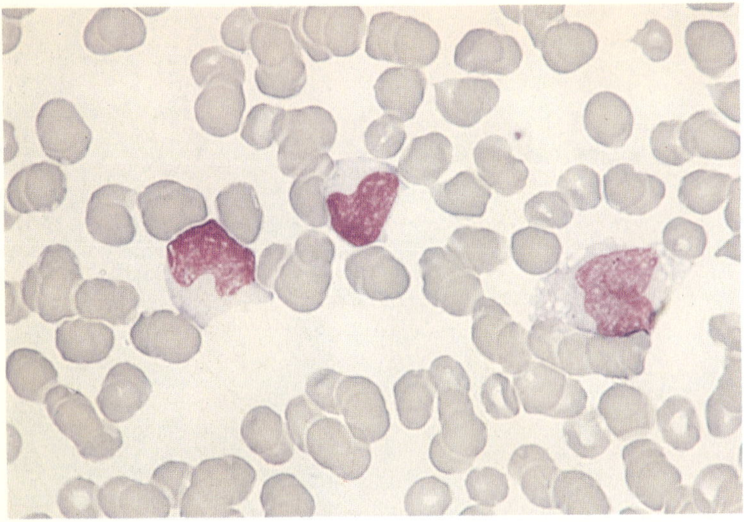

The peripheral blood from an 18-year-old girl with fever, sore throat and swollen sore eyelids is shown above.

What is the likely diagnosis?

Slide 6.11

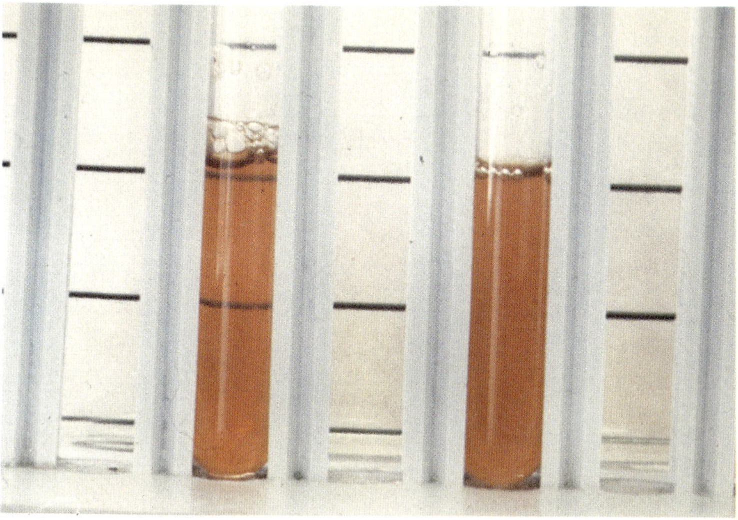

The photograph above shows a test used in the diagnosis of sickle cell disorders.

1. What is the basis of this test?
2. What other methods are available for the laboratory detection of sickle cell disorders?

Slide 6.12

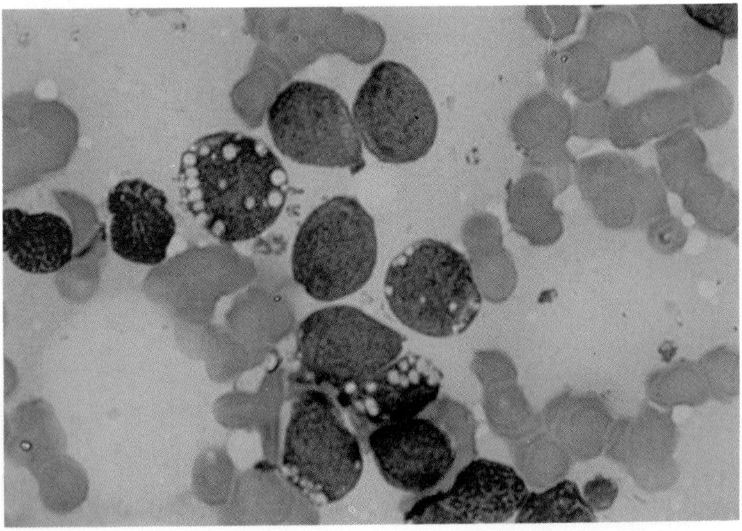

The slide above shows the bone marrow aspirate from a 7-year-old boy.

What is the differential diagnosis, and what surface marker, cytochemical, and cytogenetic characteristics would be expected?

Slide 6.13

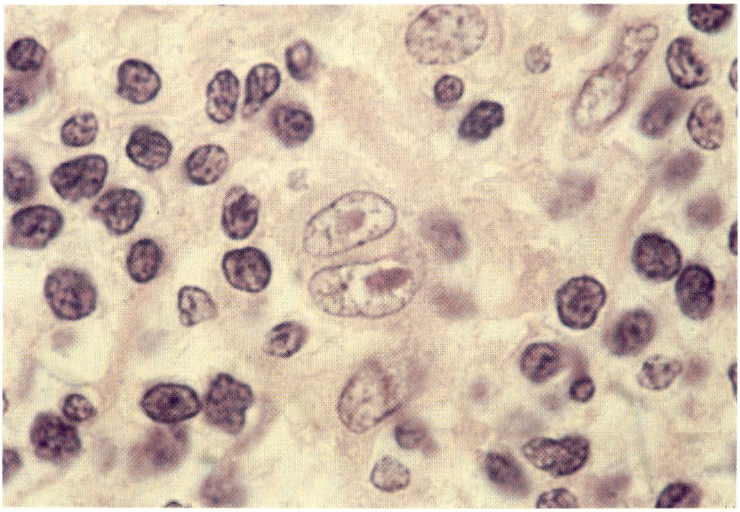

An H&E stained section of lymph node is shown above.

What is the diagnosis and what is known of the origins of the diagnostic feature shown?

Slide 6.14

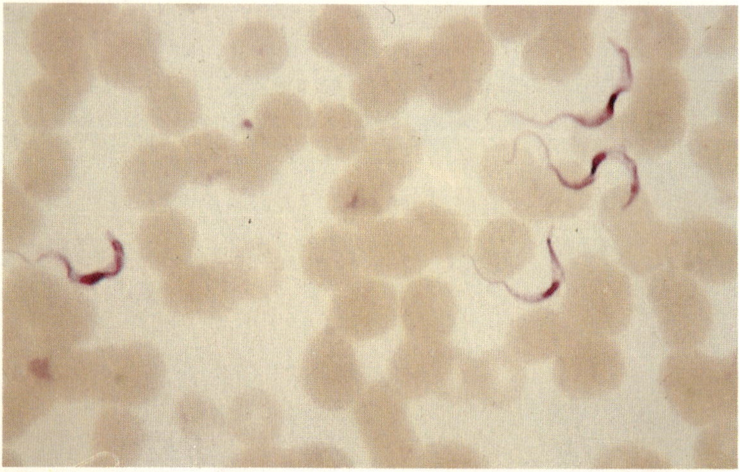

The peripheral blood from a patient with a PUO is shown above.

What is the diagnosis? How is this disease acquired?

Slide 6.15

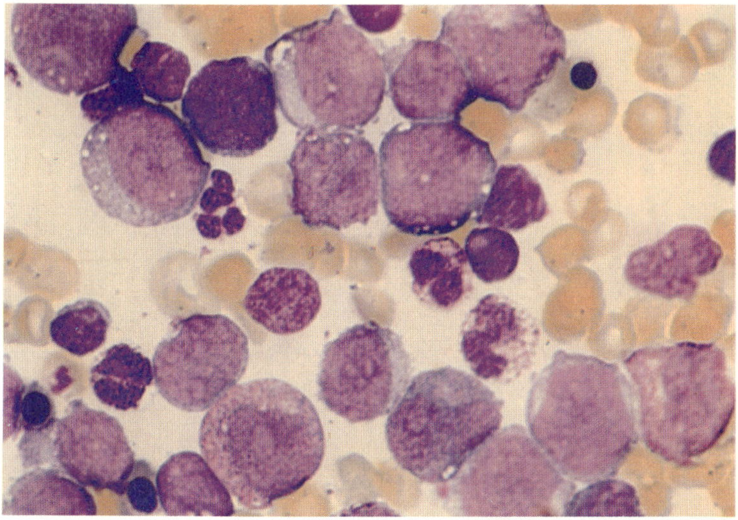

A 34-year-old-woman presented with symptoms of anaemia and menorrhagia. Blood count showed WBC 1.9 × 10^9/l, Hb 5.4 g/dl, platelets 60 × 10^9/l. Differential: neutrophils 12%, lymphocytes 71%, monocytes 4%, blasts 14%. Bone marrow aspirate is shown above.

What is the diagnosis?

Slide 6.16

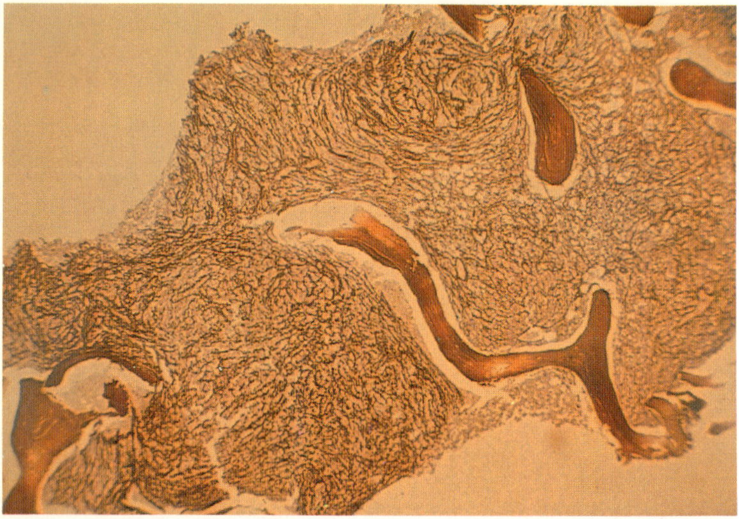

The slide above shows a trephine biopsy of bone marrow stained by silver impregnation.

What abnormality is shown and what are its causes?

Answers/Comments

Slide 6.1

The bone marrow aspirate shows two Gaucher cells. These large cells have voluminous pale crinkled cytoplasm which stains positively with PAS. They contain accumulated glucocerebroside. Inheritance of Gaucher's disease is generally autosomal recessive, and the Gaucher cells infiltrate bone marrow, spleen, liver and lymph nodes.

The pain in this case was due to a splenic infarct, revealed by ultrasound scan. These patients may also have bone pain and deformity (Erlenmeyer flask deformity).

The serum acid phosphatase is elevated, and lack of β-glucosidase in the leucocytes can be demonstrated biochemically.

Slide 6.2

This is a macrophage (reticulum cell, marrow histiocyte). It demonstrates erythrophagocytosis, with intracytoplasmic intact red cells and phagocytic vacuoles.

Histiocytic medullary reticulosis is a rare malignant proliferation of phagocytic histiocytes which is associated with erythrophagocytosis in lymph nodes and bone marrow with anaemia and hypoalbuminaemia. The malignant cell in this condition usually has a more primitive appearance than in the example shown, and this case was associated with a *Mycoplasma pneumoniae* infection. Other causes include sub-acute bacterial endocarditis and auto-immune haemolytic anaemias.

Slide 6.3

The blood film shows giant platelets with normal granule contents and the presence of a Döhle body (a blue inclusion) in the neutrophil cytoplasm. This is compatible with a diagnosis of the May-Hegglin anomaly.

Slide 6.4

The total WBC count is obviously grossly elevated and all the cells present are abnormal lymphoid cells with plentiful cytoplasm and a prominent nucleolus. The features are typical of prolymphocytic leukaemia. The majority of these disorders are of B-cell origin and the cells exhibit large amounts of surface immunoglobulin.

Slide 6.5

Megakaryocytic fragments and abnormal platelet morphology, which may be seen in acute megakaryoblastic leukaemia. This disorder overlaps with acute myelofibrosis, and a dry tap on marrow aspiration is common.

The diagnosis may be confirmed by the demonstration of platelet peroxidase by special electron microscopy techniques. The blast cells do not stain with conventional myeloperoxidase cytochemistry.

Slide 6.6

The platelet morphology of this patient shows mildly enlarged platelets which have a grey-like colour on a Romanovsky stain, and no clear granule constituents are found. This is the characteristic appearance seen in the grey platelet syndrome, which is caused by a deficiency of the α-granules. These patients occasionally have a mild bleeding tendency and there are several reports that they may develop early myelofibrosis due to defective megakaryocyte formation of platelets. This may lead to the premature release of platelet derived growth factor into the marrow environment causing excess fibroblast proliferation.

Slide 6.7

The film shows the presence of 'golf ball' inclusions of haemoglobin H in many of the red cells. The patient has HbH disease. Haemoglobin H consists of tetramers of β-chains which form because impaired α-chain production in α-thalassaemia results in a relative surplus of β-chains.

Slide 6.8

The platelets on the patient's blood film (on the left hand side) are giant platelets with an MPV of 13 fl. Further investigation by platelet aggregation revealed absent aggregation responses to 1.2 mg/ml ristocetin which was not corrected by the addition of cryoprecipitate. This is suggestive of a diagnosis of the Bernard-Soulier syndrome which can be fully substantiated by glycoprotein analysis of the platelet membrane which revealed glycoprotein Ib deficiency.

Slide 6.9

The most striking feature is a large neutrophil with very abnormal nuclear lobulation and hypogranularity. No platelets are seen. The features suggest a myelodysplastic marrow, either as a result of acute myeloid leukaemia or related to a primary myelodysplastic syndrome.

Slide 6.10

The film shows three atypical lymphocytes. The likely diagnosis in view of the history is glandular fever (infectious mononucleosis). Reactive lymphocytes demonstrate a high nuclear/cytoplasmic ratio, dark staining of the cytoplasmic edge (skirting), and indentation of the cytoplasm by surrounding red cells — 'amoeboid pseudopodia'. The nucleus may become irregular or polygonal rather than round, and sometimes the changes may be difficult to distinguish from lymphoma or acute leukaemia. The majority of reactive lymphocytes are transformed T cells reacting against EBV infected B cells.

Reactive lymphocytes may also be seen in the blood in CMV infection and other viral illnesses.

Slide 6.11

This is the sickle haemoglobin solubility test. Sickle haemoglobin is insoluble in a phosphate buffer at pH 7.1, whereas haemoglobin A remains soluble. Blood is added to the buffer, mixed and incubated. The solution goes clear pink if HbA only is present (lines on backing cards can be seen through the tube) but remains turbid if HbS is present (lines obscured). In homozygous HbSS disease centrifugation of the tube will cause the insoluble HbS to float to the surface, leaving a clear solution underneath.

Other methods for the detection of sickle haemoglobin include electrophoresis, and incubation of blood with a reducing agent such as sodium dithionite or vitamin C. After incubation at 37°C under a sealed cover slip, the red cells take up their characteristic sickled appearance.

Slide 6.12

The slide shows blast cells with fine chromatin pattern and prominent nucleoli. The cytoplasm is basophilic and contains vacuoles. The differential diagnosis is B-ALL (L3) or Burkitt lymphoma.

The vacuoles stain positively for neutral lipid (oil red O) and the cytoplasm commonly stains positively with methyl green pyronine. The cells have low TdT, are negative for acid phosphatase staining, but express common ALL antigen. Unlike common ALL, B-ALL cells express surface immunoglobulin (SIg).

One of three specific chromosomal translocations is usually found in L3 blasts: t(8:14), t(2:8), t(8:22). The segments of chromosomes involved in these translocation usually involve the immunoglobulin genes and the human oncogene c-myc is located on chromosome 8.

Approximately 2% of acute lymphoblastic leukaemias are of L3 type. They have a poorer long-term prognosis than other types of ALL. Approximately 80% of cases are male, and CNS involvement occurs in half of all cases. Hepatosplenomegaly is common and the circulating blast count is commonly low.

Slide 6.13

A binucleate giant cell with prominent nucleoli — a Reed-Sternberg (RS) cell — is shown. This is characteristic of Hodgkin's disease.

The origin of RS cells is still controversial. They may be derived from B lymphocytes but there is also evidence of macrophage origin. Many RS cells stain positively for non-specific esterase (a monocyte-macrophage characteristic). Surface and cytoplasmic immunoglobulin may be found in RS cells, but this may be derived from the ingestion of plasma immunoglobulin by a macrophage cell. RS cells have been demonstrated to possess complement C3d and immunoglobulin Fc receptors, monocyte characteristics.

Slide 6.14

The slide shows slender spindle-shaped flagellated protozoa outside the red cells — trypanosomiasis. This organism is inoculated into man by the tsetse fly, and wild game provide a reservoir of infection. The disease is characterised by fever, somnolence (hence 'sleeping sickness'), lymphadenopathy, hepatosplenomegaly and skin rashes.

Slide 6.15

The bone marrow shows increased numbers of blast cells and promyelocytes. The appearances are those of acute myeloblastic leukaemia with some differentiation of the leukaemic cells, type M2 in the FAB classification.

Slide 6.16

The marrow biopsy shows increased bone marrow reticulin — myelofibrosis. Increased reticulin is seen in the myeloproliterative disorders (myelofibrosis, polycythaemia rubra vera, essential thrombocythaemia and chronic granulocytic leukaemia), in hairy cell leukaemia, and as a reaction to marrow injury by radiation and toxic chemicals. It may also be found in disseminated tuberculosis and marrow infiltration by carcinoma or lymphoma.

In the myeloproliferative disorders fibroblast proliferation is caused by the secretion of growth factors by the megakaryocytes and platelets.

FURTHER READING

Slide 6.1
Brady R O 1972 Biochemical and metabolic basis of familial sphingolipidoses. Seminars in Hematology 9: 273
Slide 6.2
Greendyke R M et al 1963 In vitro studies on erythrophagocytosis. Blood 22: 295
Zinkham W H, Diamond L K In vitro erythrophagocytosis in acquired hemolytic anaemia. Blood 7: 592
Slide 6.3
Hamilton R W, Shaikh B S, Ottie J N, Storch J E, Saleem A, White J G 1980 Platelet function, ultrastructure, and survival in the May-Hegglin anomaly. American Journal of Clinical Pathology 74: 663
Slide 6.4
Galton D A G, Goldman J M, Wiltshaw E, Catovsky D, Henry K, Goldenberg J 1974 Prolymphocytic leukaemia. British Journal of Haematology 27: 7
Slide 6.5
Den Ottolander G J et al 1979 Megakaryoblastic leukaemia (acute myelofibrosis): a report of three cases. British Journal of Haematology 42: 9
Slide 6.6
Gerrard J M et al 1980 Biochemical studies of two patients with the gray platelet syndrome: Selective deficiency of platelet alpha granules. Journal of Clinical Investigation 66: 102
Slide 6.7
Wasi P, Na-Nakorn S, Pootrakul S 1974 The alpha thalassaemias. Clinics in Haematology 3: 383
Slide 6.8
Bithell T C, Parekh S J, Strong R R 1972 Platelet function in the Bernard-Soulier syndrome. Annals of New York Academy of Science 201: 145
Nurden A T, Caen J P 1975 Specific roles for platelet surface glycoproteins in platelet function. Nature 255: 720
Slide 6.9
Pierre R V 1974 Preleukemic states. Seminars in Hematology 11: 73
Slide 6.10
Wood T A, Frenkel E P 1967 The atypical lymphocyte. American Journal of Medicine 42: 923
Slide 6.11
Huntsman R G, Barclay G P T, Canning G M, Dawson G I 1970 A rapid whole blood solubility test to differentiate the sickle-cell trait from sickle-cell anaemia. Journal of Clinical Pathology 23: 781
Slide 6.12
Greaves M F 1981 Analysis of the clinical and biological significance of lymphoid phenotypes in acute leukaemia. Cancer Research 41: 4752
Jackson P F et al 1982 Cytogenetics of B-cell lineage acute lymphocytic leukaemias of childhood. Lancet ii: 1334
Rowley J D 1982 Identification of the constant chromosome regions involved in human hematologic malignant disease. Science 216: 749
Slide 6.13
Káplan H S, Gartner S 1977 'Sternberg-Reed' giant cells of Hodgkin's disease: Cultivation in vitro, heterotransplantation, and characterisation as neoplastic macrophages. International Journal of Cancer 19: 511
Order S E, Hellman S 1972 Pathogenesis of Hodgkin's disease. Lancet i: 571

Slide 6.14
Wery M et al 1982 Hematologic manifestations, diagnosis and immunopathology of African trypanosomiasis. Seminars in Hematology 19: 83

Slide 6.15
Bennett J M et al 1976 Proposals for the classification of the acute leukaemias. British Journal of Haematology 33: 451

Slide 6.16
Jacobson R S, Salo A, Fialkow P S 1978 Agnogenic myeloid metaplasia: A clonal proliferation of hematopoietic stem cells with secondary myelofibrosis. Blood 51: 189

Index

The page numbers in parentheses refer to answers